THE DECIMATION OF U.S. HEALTHCARE

Copyright © 2025 James E. Harper. All rights reserved.

Copyright Registration number: TXu 2-479-110
Library of Congress Control Number: 2025910093
ISBN: 9798998780516

No part of this book may be reproduced, distributed, or transmitted in any form or by any means, including photocopying, recording, or other electronic or mechanical methods, without the prior written permission of the publisher, except in the case of brief quotations embodied in critical reviews and specific other noncommercial uses permitted by copyright law.

Table of Contents

Foreword 1

Chapter 1: The Beginning of Rushed Doctor Visits 3

Chapter 2: A Giant Grows 6

Chapter 3: How the Giant Was Able to Grow So Big 11

Chapter 4: Who Has Suffered the Most from the Trampling of the Giant? 16

Chapter 5: The Creation of a Monster—A Legalized Scam 21

Chapter 6: The Plot Thickens 28

Chapter 7: Primary Care Physicians, Small Hospitals and Clinics: How the Backbone Was Broken 40

Chapter 8: A Failing Health Care System: Is There Any Hope for A Revival? 62

Chapter 9: The Root of The Evil and Perhaps the Way Out 68

References 100

Foreword

When I was growing up, I admired TV Doctors like Dr. Kildare and Marcus Welby MD. Why? Because they seemed intelligent, reliable, empathetic, and patient. I also thought they seemed like heroes and I wanted to grow up to be like that. These are qualities that everyone wants their doctor to have. Of course, everyone realizes that a doctor is human and therefore, imperfect. However, much is expected of a doctor after so many years of education and training. Since the US is the richest country in the world, it would be expected to have the best health care system in the world. Yet, the facts show exactly the opposite. The US spends more on health care than any other country in the world, but at the same time has one of the worst health care outcomes in the world. In fact, in 2022 US healthcare cost 4.5 trillion dollars with an average of $13,493 per person. (1) By comparison, the average healthcare cost per person in other wealthy countries is less than half as much. How could this be? What happened that resulted in this debacle?

To answer these questions, we must go back to the beginning of the problem and note how it developed. Third-party entities played an early role between the doctor and the patient. Indeed, private insurance companies have been operative since the early 1900s. But, a turning point in their pivotal role was yet to come. On July 30, 1965, President Lyndon B. Johnson signed the Medicare and Medicaid Act, also known as the Social Security Amendment of 1965, into law. It established Medicare, a health insurance program for the elderly, and Medicaid, a health insurance program for people with limited income. (2) These were government programs funded by taxpayer dollars with the ultimate goal of improving the healthcare disparity in the US. In the beginning, these programs filled in the medical gaps for the disabled, the elderly, and the poor. But things happened to change this objective. These events will be outlined in this book as well as the consequences of doing so.

Chapter 1: The Beginning of Rushed Doctor Visits

Many people now tell me that their previous doctor 'was in and out'. They recall briefly talking to the doctor, who rushed out stating "I will order labs, and "Have a great rest of your day". Many times, this occurs without any semblance of an examination. When and how did this dubious practice begin?

Analysts feel that the origin of the rushed doctor visits came about in 1992, when Medicare adopted a bizarre formula that relied on "relative value units" or RVUs, to calculate doctor's fees. The typical office visit for a primary care patient was said to be 1.3 RVUs and the AMA coding guidelines for that type of visit suggested a 15-minute consult. (3) No longer was a doctor given credit for the time he spent with a patient or the time spent arriving at the correct diagnosis and treatment. A doctor's time involved in unraveling a complex condition that a patient suffered from no longer had any value. The most important thing was to see patients as quickly as possible, no matter what their problem was. This system led to devaluing the cognitive aspect of care rendered by a physician to their patient about evaluating and managing their condition. Also, there was no further adjustment of value when taking into account the doctor's education, training, and experience.

Primary Care Providers were hit the hardest since insurance companies lump them into one category: Physician Assistants, Nurse Practitioners, General Practitioners, Family Practitioners, and physicians specializing in Internal Medicine, even though the level of education and training is entirely different for each of these professions. Private insurers, in turn, jumped on the bandwagon and quickly copied Medicare's fee schedule.

THE DECIMATION OF U.S. HEALTHCARE

This new system dictated that all physicians, whether considered primary care or "specialists" had to be 'in and out' with a patient. The reason is because if they spent more time, they would not be compensated for the visit. This huge decline in compensation is in stark contrast to lawyers, accountants, and engineers as well as other professionals who can set their hourly rate according to their level of education and expertise and they thoroughly expect to receive it. Also, these professions are not relegated to receive compensation by either government programs or by profiteering insurance companies. Physicians are not only subjected to these conditions but are also obligated to accept huge discounts from their standard charges.

This momentous change in the physician's venue gave impetus to the already emerging "managed care" that took over the healthcare industry shortly thereafter. Doctors, who participated in managed care networks, had to sign contracts that gave huge discounts on their previous service rates. In exchange, the third-party private insurers promised to steer patients to them and to pay claims promptly. But the reality has been quite different. As a result of private insurers and managed care contracts' drastic reduction of compensation, doctors were forced to increase daily patient volumes to maintain stable incomes. This fee-for-service system has left primary care physicians feeling as though they were in an assembly line rather than caring for patients compassionately and thoughtfully. No doubt, this factors into the current severe shortage of primary care physicians that we currently have.

The situation is compounded by the fact that while the inflation rate and cost of living have steadily risen, the Medicare fee-for-service rates have not kept pace. Annual updates to prices are set through statute and regulation. These prices have risen by less than 0.5% a year since 2015.

THE DECIMATION OF U.S. HEALTHCARE

Despite the highest inflation rate in almost 40 years in 2023, Medicare cut its rate to physician providers in 2024 by 3.4%(4) In addition, Medicare offers payment rates to providers on a 'take it or leave it' basis. Providers who do not want to accept these rates can decline to participate. However, this is not a feasible option for most physicians. Why? Because Medicare accounts for such a large share of US healthcare spending. To walk away from it would be suicide for a practice. Therefore, physicians who have small clinics or smaller hospitals would have no financial ability to opt out of the program. It is clear why private corporate giants are taking over hospitals and small clinics.

Another reason why Medicare prices usually trend lower is due to the fact that Medicare is a federal program which is funded by tax payer dollars. Since Medicare is required to achieve budget neutrality annually, physicians are usually the objects of pay cuts. Indeed, Medicare is mainly funded by payroll taxes. This means that any proposal to raise its spending must be financed through higher taxes or premiums, which translates into increases in federal debt or cuts in Medicare benefits or other spending. Private plans have been part of Medicare since the year after its beginning in 1966. (5). However, something happened in 1997 that changed the landscape of the healthcare industry. This will be discussed in the next chapter.

Chapter 2: A Giant Grows

The Balanced Budget Act of 1997 initiated Medicare Part C which later became known as Medicare Advantage Plans. Also, PPOs (Preferred Provider Organizations) were established to allow beneficiaries the option to obtain services and providers outside of the provider network. This was in contrast to the already existing HMOs (Health Maintenance Organizations), which only permitted access to providers and services within the network. Medicare Advantage became the alias name of the privatized portion of Medicare run primarily by major insurance companies. These plans generally offer extra benefits, such as eyeglasses and dental care, not available under original Medicare. Medicare Advantage plans argue that most seniors are pleased with these plans versus traditional Medicare.

You may ask the question: Why and how did a federal program become in part, privatized? As is true of so many altruistic initiatives, the intentions were wholesome and pure in the beginning. The original purpose was to give Medicare beneficiaries the choice of access to well-managed care at a lower cost. However, quite the opposite has occurred. Medicare Advantage has expanded to encompass more than half of all Medicare beneficiaries and costs far more per beneficiary than traditional Medicare ever has. In fact, according to some health services research, Medicare Advantage will cost Medicare over $600 billion more in the next eight years from 2023 to 2031 than would have been expected if the same enrollees had remained in traditional Medicare. Also, the evidence is in favor of the conclusion that Medicare Advantage enrollees neither receive better care nor do they have better health outcomes.

What is the financial relationship between Medicare and Medicare Advantage plans? Medicare Advantage plans are private insurance plans that receive monthly funding based on a coding system from Medicare and premiums charged to their enrollees. In contrast, medical providers bill original Medicare for each service provided. The way it works is that the federal government pays private insurers, not medical practitioners, a fixed amount per month for each patient, based on their risk of getting sick, called a capitated amount. The amount depends on an assessment of the beneficiaries' medical records and the expected healthcare costs in the county in which they live. Higher rates are paid for sicker patients and less is paid for those in good health. This means that the more serious medical conditions "the plans" diagnose, the more money the "plan", not the medical practitioner, gets. These "plans" can receive thousands of dollars more per patient than is justified with little monitoring by the Center for Medicare Services (CMS).

Since Medicare Advantage plans are a form of "managed care", their main objective is to spend as little as possible on patient care to maintain a high-profit margin. They do this by imposing strict regulations on services provided and on whether or not claims will be paid to providers of these services as well as to how much will be paid for these services. One of the methods employed is Utilization Management. This includes preadmission certification and concurrent review of hospital admissions. So-called "gatekeepers," primary care providers, were supposed to limit access of patients to specialists. Another method of restraint imposed by Medicare Advantage plans is the requirement for prior authorization for medications or referrals to see specialists. Neither of these methods has improved care. The contrary has been true. Care has been critically delayed and, in some cases, denied. As expected, all this has been to the detriment and in some cases, to the demise of the patient. This has also led to the gradual disappearance of small clinics and even small hospitals. In fact, instead of lone doctors working in private practice, physicians have been forced to consolidate by joining large medical groups. Hospitals were closing in the late 1990s and many more were forced to join hospital systems to survive. Between 1990 and 2000, there were more than 100 hospital mergers in the U.S..(6).

What have been the financial results of these Medicare Advantage plans? It has been a tale of two stories. The cost of insuring Medicare beneficiaries through Medicare Advantage was 22% to 35% higher or between $88 billion to $140 billion more than it would have been had those beneficiaries remained in traditional Medicare. On the flip side, the Medicare Advantage Plans have rocketed to become by far the most profitable branches of large insurance companies. Medicare Advantage plans have become a parasite within Medicare in that these plans are not only surviving within Medicare, but they are also flourishing, raking in huge profits as a result of this symbiotic relationship. For example, United Health Group had a record of $17.3 billion in profit in 2021. (7) Yet, in 2022, United Health Group made over $20.6 billion in profit. (8).

To put this into perspective, all of America's largest insurers collectively made more than $41 billion in profit in 2022. Therefore, one health insurer made almost half that much in profit. United Health Group made a whopping $324 billion in revenues in 2023. Only Walmart, Amazon, Apple, and Exxon Mobil exceeded their earnings in that year. There is no doubt that with regard to the latching on of Medicare Advantage Plans to Medicare, a taxpayer-funded federal program, corporate greed is alive and well in America. In fact, of the 10 highest-paid healthcare executives in the US in 2020, three were from Oak Street Health, with salary and benefits amounting to 568 million for the CEO. Of course, executives in large hospitals commonly have salaries and benefits to the tune of several million dollars a year.

What is the main difference between traditional Medicare and Medicare Advantage plans? Medicare is mainly funded by payroll taxes. For example, the amount in 2019 was $12,000 per year not including Part D expenses. Also, the traditional Medicare program does not channel money through insurance companies. Instead, it pays doctors and hospitals directly. Moreover, it devotes around 2% of its expenditures to administrative costs. To the delight of doctors and hospitals, Medicare pays claims promptly usually responding within a 15-day time frame. Furthermore, Medicare, as opposed to Medicare Advantage plans does not deny claims alleging lack of medical necessity.

In contrast, Medicare Advantage plans are heavily burdened with administrative fees. Some research shows that health insurance companies take 15% of the money received from Medicare which is taxpayer-funded to pay for their administrative costs and profit before directing the other 85% to doctors and hospitals for payment of their respective services. This fact sheds some light on why doctors and hospitals have to accept such deep discounts from their original charges for such services provided. In other words, doctors and hospitals are suffering ever-increasing losses while health insurance companies are reaping huge profits through Medicare Advantage plans at everyone else's expense. Other studies show an even more grim picture. It is estimated that only 60% of the health care dollars spent annually in the US go toward medical care. That is, in paying doctors and hospitals for services provided. Physicians only accounted for 10% of U.S. healthcare spending. Probably at least 34% of the health care dollars spent per annum goes toward billing, marketing, and yes, you guessed it, insurance company profits and administrative costs. Indeed, one study showed that approximately 15% of U.S. healthcare spending is due to higher administrative costs associated with health insurance. This includes costs related to eligibility, coding, submission, and rework. Another 15% of U.S. healthcare spending is also due to the administrative burden on providers largely from insurance companies, general administration, human resources, quality reporting, and accreditation. (9) Even so, this menace to US healthcare grew larger. How? This will be discussed in the next chapter.

Chapter 3: How the Giant Was Able to Grow So Big

Some may reason that the health insurance companies must have shrewd businessmen working for them to become so profitable. This is true. But, being shrewd does not equate with honesty or integrity. Far from it. The health insurance industry uses unscrupulous means to maintain their profits higher and higher. How? One way is by denying legitimate claims by doctors and hospitals. For example, after a doctor evaluates a patient in a clinic or hospital setting, the doctor or the billing department submits a claim to the respective insurance company for payment of the services, irrespective of co-pays received in advance.

The insurance companies are supposed to evaluate the claim and respond promptly. Unfortunately, this is not what happens in most cases. Many health insurance companies who claim to provide medical care for their enrollees either deny to pay the claims, grossly underpay the claims that are already deeply discounted or falsely claim to pay the claims to providers, most of whom are doctors. For example, UnitedHealthcare denies 32%, almost one-third of the claims submitted to them. The most common reason cited is the lack of medical necessity. So, essentially what they are alleging is that the patient had no right to see the doctor and that the doctor should have refused to see the patient despite their physical complaints. Other top insurance companies also have high denial rates including Anthem Blue Cross Blue Shield at 23% and Aetna at 20%. Other reasons for denial include missed deadlines or policy exclusions. (10)

One strategy frequently used by health insurance companies is to rigidly deny broad categories or types of claims without taking the time to evaluate whether the specific claim is covered under their plan or policy.

The insurer plays the "ignorant game" and deliberately avoids learning the facts in hopes that the claim will be dropped or the time for refiling a claim will expire. Another tactic is that insurers employ auditing software programmed to deny claims instantly because the ultimate goal is to limit payouts to doctors and hospitals. Many of these auditing programs work by finding technical errors in billing codes that all doctors and hospitals submit for payment.

A notorious example of the use of this malware is Cigna. This health insurance company has built a system that instantly rejects claims without opening the patient file, leaving people with unexpected bills from the doctor or hospital and leaving both groups unpaid. It has been reported that Cigna personnel, alleged to be "doctors", denied over 300,000 requests for payments using this method. The time spent in each case was on average an astonishing 1.2 seconds per request! Cigna claims to provide health care plans for 18 million people in the US. Supposedly, most state laws and regulations require insurance companies to have company doctors review claims before rejecting them. Many states require the medical director of insurance companies to examine patient records, review coverage policies, and use their medical expertise to decide whether to approve or deny claims.

But Cigna utilizes an algorithm that flags mismatches between diagnoses and what the company has programmed the software to be acceptable which includes tests and procedures for these conditions. Mismatches are instantaneously rejected and company doctors then sign off on these denials. (11). Cigna has perpetuated this dubious system without much concern about whether or not it is lawful. The company has been employing this same software system for over a decade. In contrast, both Medicare and Medicaid have a software system that prevents payment of claims that are incorrectly coded. However, it does not reject payment on medical grounds.

Unfortunately, health insurance companies may use any of many other tactics to reduce payments to doctors and hospitals to secure their profits. The result is that the bill is either passed on to the patient or the doctors and/or hospitals suffer the loss. These tactics fall under the broad category of Bad Faith. They include misrepresentation which refers to providing false information regarding coverage. Underpayment is a frequent tactic which is when the insurance company tries to pay a claim at a lower amount than is advertised and/or expected. The insurance company may also refuse to pay the doctor or provider for the extra time submitted to manage the patient without explanation. For example, insurance companies are supposed to pay above the Medicare rate which has been reduced consistently every year for the last 20 years.

According to a report by the Congressional Budget Office for physician services overall, commercial insurers paid on average 129% of Medicare Fee For Service prices between 2010-2020 ranging from 118%-163% depending on the specialty and service provided. Unfortunately, primary care services or office visits during this time were paid at the lowest rate averaging 117% of Medicare Fee For Service, while specialist services were paid at a rate of 144% of Medicare Fee For Service. As previously mentioned, primary care is lumped together with mid-level practitioners like physician assistants and nurse practitioners, general practitioners who have one year of internship after medical school, family practitioners who must have a three-year residency of broad training after medical school, and Internal Medicine doctors who undergo a three-year residency training in the specialty of Internal Medicine after medical school. Yet, all these practitioners, despite their vast differences in training and education, are paid at the same rate by the insurance companies, distinct from so-called "specialists". Another tactic employed is a lack of explanation. This involves failing to give a complete or valid justification when denying a claim. This method is commonly used to delay claim requests past the expiration date.

A further bad faith tactic is failure to disclose. This refers to an insurance company not informing a client or provider what coverage applies to a specific payment. The plea of ignorance encompasses failure to investigate. This tactic involves a refusal to pay a claim without a reasonable investigation. The example of Cigna is noteworthy. Additionally, health insurers submit incredibly complex contracts for doctors and other providers to sign, purposely omitting details like specific fee schedules for various medical billing codes to deceive the signing party. All of these practices by health insurance companies have the objective to avoid payment of a claim or to reduce the size of the claim. The ultimate goal of the third-party private health insurer is to reduce costs and increase profits. (12)

Are there laws and regulations to stop these unfair practices of health insurance companies? Unfortunately, the few laws that exist are skimpy and vague at best which explains why the health insurance companies are blatantly operating in a rogue fashion. Especially vulnerable, are small primary care clinics with single physicians, as well as small hospitals. This, in large part, explains why there is an incredible shortage of physicians in the US, most notably among so-called primary care providers. The insurance companies know that there are few options for the victims of their lawlessness, whether it be a physician or a patient. Most states have an insurance commissioner usually located at the capitol of the respective state whom someone can file complaints against the particular insurance company. However, it is highly questionable as to whether anything will be done about it or even if the insurance company will be disciplined or regulated in any way.

Even the Center for Medicare Services has no mechanism to regulate or censure the health insurers involved in Medicare Advantage plans. No doubt, this is also the reason why many doctors have opted to no longer accept various health insurance policies or to become entirely independent of health insurance by accepting cash or credit card payments only. In short, the politicians have failed to control the giant health insurers which have made a fortune off Medicare, a tax payer funded federal program. They are swallowing up doctors, other nonphysician providers, and hospitals in their path in an unimpeded effort to become as rich as possible, all with the full blessing and support of US lawmakers. But who are the main victims of this stampede for wealth in the healthcare industry? The answer to this question and more will be discussed in the next chapter.

Chapter 4: Who Has Suffered the Most from the Trampling of the Giant?

As the US population grows and ages and the physician shortage is ever increasing, we are moving ever closer toward a perfect storm. It is projected that by 2035, there will be more seniors aged 65 and over than there will be children aged 17 or younger. That will be a demographic milestone this nation has never reached. (13). The trend is obvious. The US population aged 65 and over grew nearly five times as fast as the total population over the 100 years from 1920 to 2020. About 1 in 6 people in the US were age 65 and over in 2020 compared to only 1 in 20 in 1920. The older population increased by 50.9 million, from 4.9 million (4.7%) of the US population in 1920 to 55.8 million (16.8%)of the US population in 2020. This represents a growth rate of about 1000%, almost five times that of the total population (about 200%). The trend is also accelerating. In the 10 years between 2010 and 2020, the 65 and over population in the US saw its largest-ever numeric gain with an increase of 15.5 million people. (14).

What is the current situation about the aging population and what are the projections for the near future? As of 2022, there were 57.8 million adults age 65 and over living in the US. (15). By 2036, the US population is projected to grow by 8.4%. Furthermore, the population aged 65 and over is projected to grow an astonishing 34.1% with an even more surprising increase of 54.7% in the size of the population of those persons 75 and older. (16) What does this mean for the healthcare system in the US? An older population means an increase in the prevalence of more chronic diseases. An aging population tends to require more health care and access to more physicians. This trend will lead to an ever-increasing demand for physicians.

The ten most prevalent and costly chronic diseases in the US currently are the following: obesity, hypertension, high cholesterol, coronary artery disease, asthma, chronic kidney disease, diabetes, cancer (excluding skin cancer), and depression. (17) This means there is a greater need for more doctors, especially primary care doctors who routinely evaluate and manage patients with these chronic diseases. Primary care physicians include pediatricians, general practitioners, family practitioners and doctors specialized in Internal Medicine. Indeed, Internal Medicine physicians are uniquely trained to care for the chronic medical problems of adolescents and adults while Pediatricians are uniquely trained to care for the chronic medical problems of infants and children.

What are the expectations on the horizon for physicians to meet these demands? Physicians currently age 65 and older make up 20% of the clinical physician workforce and those between ages 55-64 make up 22% of the clinical physician workforce. This means that a significant number of physicians in the US are currently at or nearing retirement age. Furthermore, the total projected shortage of physicians in the US by 2036 is between 13,500 and 86,000. The projections for primary care physicians are even more ominous. The projected shortage of primary care physicians in the US by 2036 is between 20,200 and 40,400. (18)

What accounts for such great physician shortages? One recent survey based on 1,639 doctors gave the five following reasons: 1) Burnout accounting for 59%. Physicians do not feel valued at their work. There may be cultural or management concerns. There may be a lack of support for their well-being. An example of this is the increased security risks for physicians in the workplace, particularly in hospitals, emergency departments, and even clinics due to gun violence. Increasingly, doctors, other medical providers, and hospitals are becoming the targets of gun violence. Another reason is that the work-life balance may not balance with the needs of the physician. Also, many physicians have to work long hours.

2) Moral injury accounts for 16%. Physicians are forced to consider factors other than medical judgment when determining a patient's treatment. There may be widespread corporate violations. They may have to deal with a lack of autonomy as a result of this "managed care" system in which insurance companies frequently dictate care patterns. 3) Cost of living/inflation concerns account for 9%. Physicians must constantly balance their work location with their potential compensation or higher compensation due to their cost of living and if they have a private practice, their overhead costs. In the year 2023, inflation was reportedly higher than in the previous 40-50 years. 4) Corporate advancement/benefits accounts for 5%. Physicians are leaving their jobs for better positions, career advancement, and non-clinical roles. In 2021, 117,000 physicians left the practice of medicine.

This mass exodus was, no doubt, in part due to issues connected to the COVID-19 pandemic. As of 2023, more doctors moved into healthcare administration, technologic, pharmaceuticals and medical writing sectors. 5) Family concerns account for 5%. The explanation was not enough opportunities or time for spouse and children and a desire to be closer to family members. (19)

Another study mentioned some of the biggest reasons for physician burnout driving them to leave the practice of medicine include: ongoing physician shortages, system inefficiencies, administrative burdens, and increasing regulatory and technological requirements. 81% of physicians feel overworked while 88% say the existing shortage negatively impacts their practice. Low pay coupled with high workloads and a labor shortage all contribute to burnout and an ever-worsening shortage of physicians in the US.(20)

The most critical area of physician shortage in the US is primary care. One report projects a shortage of 68,020 full-time primary care physicians by 2036. Why is primary care so important to the health care system? A primary care physician is often the first contact a patient will have with the health care workforce and sets into motion whether the patient will have a positive or negative experience as well as their outcome. A high-functioning primary care system not only treats illnesses and injuries before these become severe but also provides ongoing care to achieve the optimal outcome for chronic conditions.

A good primary care physician will refer to more specialized care when it is required and will select the most qualified subspecialists needed for the particular problem the patient is facing.(21). Primary care is the backbone of the health care system. It is the only area in which the services result in better population health and more equitable outcomes. Without primary care, minor health problems can quickly spiral into a chronic disease, with poor disease management and emergency room overuse along with unsustainable costs. Several studies have shown that primary care services may be associated with lower total healthcare expenditures. A recent study found that the average annual total cost of the patients having a primary care provider was 27.4% lower than those without a primary care provider.(22). So, the conclusion is clear: Primary care not only leads to better health outcomes and overall greater equity in health care access, but it also results in lower per capita health care costs. Therefore, primary care is essential for a well-functioning healthcare system.

However, the facts show that primary care physicians in the US are disappearing rapidly. In 1980, 62% of doctor's visits for adults 65 and over were for primary care and 38% were for specialists. By 2013, this ratio was reversed and now the situation is much worse. We now have a specialty-driven healthcare system. Currently, only about 25% of US doctors are in primary care. This means that more than 100 million Americans don't have regular access to primary care. This figure has more than doubled since 2014. No wonder the US ranks last among wealthy countries in certain healthcare outcomes. Even the average life span in America is decreasing while it is increasing in many other countries. (23). What is the primary reason for this physician crisis? This will be discussed in the next chapter.

Chapter 5: The Creation of a Monster—A Legalized Scam

As mentioned previously in an earlier chapter, health insurance companies have been operating in the US since the early 1900s. A big win for private insurers came in 1954 when Congress enacted legislation that exempted employer-sponsored health insurance from federal income taxation. The tax code effectively encouraged employees and their employers to shift compensation toward untaxed health insurance and away from taxed money income. To put this into perspective, the Congressional Budget Office estimated that the federal tax subsidy alone amounted to almost $250 billion in 2013, most of which went into the pockets of third-party private insurers. The entire spending for Medicare for both inpatient and outpatient services in 2012 was only slightly less. (24).

The birth of Medicare and Medicaid came in 1965. On July 30.1965, President Lyndon B. Johnson signed the Medicare and Medicaid Act, also known as the Social Security Amendment of 1965. This law established Medicare as a health insurance program for the elderly while Medicaid was proposed to be a health insurance program for people with limited income. As is true with so many well-intentioned plans in the beginning, the results usually end up far from the goal.

From Medicare's inception in 1965 until 1992, physicians set charge rates for the medical care they provided to patients. Medicare reined in price uniformity by using a CPR (Customary, Prevailing, and Reasonable) charge system. This was adopted from the Usual, Customary, and Reasonable (UCR) system that was used by private insurers. In this CPR system, Medicare defined customary charges as the median of a physician's charges for a given service. The prevailing charge was initially set at the 90th percentile of the customary charges of all same specialties physicians in a region. Medicare went on to define the reasonable charge as the lowest of payments received for a customary charge or the prevailing charge in the Medicare payment area. Are you confused yet? As you have likely discerned, there were problems with this method.

One of the problems was that charges for the same service under the CPR system led to considerable variation in physician compensation. Another problem was that individual Medicare carriers with various policies resulted in huge disparities in physician compensation. For example, some carriers paid all providers one prevailing charge for a service while others paid each specialty physician a different prevailing rate for that service. Another point of controversy was that CPR regulations were unable to prevent physicians from raising their fees.

Thus, the (CMS) Center for Medicare Services stepped in to control Medicare costs by decreasing the prevailing charge from the 90th to the 75th percentile. However, this decision disregarded rising physician costs associated with changes in clinical practice and technology. As a result, compensation for office visits failed to keep pace with the increased physician overhead brought about due to changes in economic trends as well as the increasing complexity and cost associated with diagnosing and managing patients. Rural physicians were especially hard hit, with their compensation held to the prevailing charges of the 1970s despite technological advancements. (25) So with all of these challenges, something had to change.

THE DECIMATION OF U.S. HEALTHCARE

In 1992, a monumental change in Medicare was instituted. Medicare adopted a system called RVUs (Relative Value Units) to calculate physician payments, as an effort to create a standardized physician fee schedule. RVUs that were assigned to a procedure or service compared its value relative to other procedures or services. For example, if a service had 6 total RVUs, this meant the resources consumed in delivering that service were 6 times greater than those consumed by a procedure with 1 RVU. Various types of RVUs were then created.

Work RVUs take into consideration a provider's work involved with performing a procedure or service. Variables used to determine this value include technical skills, physical effort, mental effort, and judgment, along with the stress related to patient risk and the amount of time required to perform the service or procedure. Practice expense RVUs were created to reflect the cost of clinical and nonclinical labor and expenses of the provider's practice. This was proposed to include medical supplies, office supplies, clinical and administrative staff as well as prorate costs of building space, utilities, medical equipment, and office equipment. Malpractice RVUs were developed to reflect the cost of professional liability insurance based on an estimate of the relative risk associated with each CPT code a physician is accustomed to using. How is this consideration of the value of a physician's work translated to a dollar figure? Also, how is the mental effort of a physician or other medical practitioner quantified for payment purposes?

What is employed is the so-called MPF (Medicare Physician Fee) Conversion Factor. The conversion factor is an arbitrary dollar figure selected which is multiplied by the RVU to determine the physician payment schedule. The dollar conversion factor has been steadily shrinking for physicians over the previous years. For example, the conversion factor for 2020 was $36.089, 2021 $34.8931, 2022 $34.6062, 2023 $33.8872 and 2024 $32.7442. But this is not the only way the Medicare Physician Fee Schedule is determined. The calculation is much more complex. The following is the so-called basic formula used by Medicare to determine physician compensation for codes on the MPFS (Medicare Physician Fee Schedule where GPCI represents Geographic Practice Cost Indices: [(Work RVU x Work GPCI) +(PE RVU x PE GPCI) +(MP RVU x MP GPCI)] x CF = payment amount. (26). No wonder that private insurers quickly adopted Medicare's Physician Fee Schedule seeing this as a way to pay physicians and other health care providers significantly less while simultaneously reaping huge profits by steadily raising their annual premiums.

Since its inception, Medicare has traditionally rewarded surgical subspecialties who perform surgery as well as medical subspecialties who perform procedures with much higher compensation compared to primary care physicians including Internal Medicine physicians, Family Practice physicians, General Practice physicians, and Pediatricians. As time has gone on, the disparity has become even greater. Many experts feel that the origin of the rushed 15-minute primary care doctor which has become the "norm" arose as a result of Medicare's adoption of this formula that relies on RVUs (Relative Value Units). The AMA initially coupled with Medicare to create this rushed visit. Medicare came up with the figure of 1.3 RVUs which was said to be the value of a typical office visit for a primary care patient.

According to the AMA coding guidelines, that type of visit suggested a fifteen-minute consult. Private insurers immediately piggybacked this move by only paying for 15 minutes of a physician's time even though a patient consultation usually takes much more of the physician's time. (27). This explains why private insurers and Medicare will only pay for about 15 minutes of the doctor's time for a physical examination which is supposed to be a comprehensive annual assessment of the patient. This should include a detailed history of current symptoms, review of systems and family history in addition to the physical examination. An evaluation of this caliber is next to impossible to fit into 15 minutes which is why most physicians punt and merely tell the patient that they will order lab work. Also, other factors that were supposed to be considered in physician compensation, especially with regard to primary care physicians, were left out. This new development, along with private insurers dominating the health care system and with the advent of "managed care," struck a serious blow to physicians, particularly those involved in primary care.

Third-party private health insurers required physicians to participate in "managed care" networks where they were obligated to agree to give insured patients large discounts on their rates. In turn, the insurer promised to pay the physician promptly and to continue to steer patients their way. However, there was no accounting for the cognitive and communicative skills needed by a primary care physician to evaluate and manage patients nor for the time and effort involved. For example, a primary care physician must spend time evaluating a patient which involves direct patient care including history taking, physical examination, explaining the patient's condition or the possibilities given a complex case, and explaining recommendations or answering the questions of a patient.

Also, indirect patient care is involved, such as answering e-mails, telephone calls, reviewing labs, imaging studies, discussing a patient's management with colleagues or spending time to make referrals to other providers on behalf of the patient. Gone are the days of a long methodical doctor visit when a physician could thoughtfully take a detailed history, perform an equally detailed physical exam to arrive at the correct diagnosis, or provide the best screening tests in the case of a preventative health exam. It seems that the physician has been forced to rapidly move patients in and out to survive. This means physicians have to make quicker decisions regarding diagnosis and treatment which no doubt has led to a greater likelihood of clinical errors. A primary care physician's time to take care of a patient is no longer taken into account. This is in stark contrast with other professions including lawyers or accountants who charge fixed hourly rates and are thus compensated for the time spent serving their clients.

The disparity was even greater for primary care physicians with the adoption of the RVU system by Medicare and private insurers to determine compensation for physicians. RVUs were created for surgical subspecialties and medical subspecialties involved with procedures. However, no significant adjustment was made for the primary care visit despite the rapid evolution of medical science and technology, not to mention physician practice overhead expenses. Primary care physicians had no other option but to markedly increase their daily patient volume while at the same time decreasing the time spent with each patient to maintain their income levels. This caused a perpetual cycle of physicians feeling as though they were working on an assembly line rather than engaged in a mission to heal the sick and prevent serious illness. (28)

A decisive blow was made to the US healthcare system in 1997. The Balanced Budget Act of 1997 was passed by Congress initiating Medicare Part C which became known as Medicare Advantage Plans. These plans received payments from Medicare which is primarily funded by payroll taxes. (29). More specifically, Medicare is financed by two Trust Funds. A Hospital Insurance Trust Fund finances Medicare Part A which is primarily financed through payroll taxes on US workers and employees. A Supplementary Medical Insurance trust fund supports Part A and Part D. Part D provides prescription coverage for Medicare beneficiaries. Most of the financing comes from the US federal government's general fund because premiums only cover about 1/4 of the fund's total expenditures.

Part C which is the Medicare Advantage Plans are paid for by the Hospital Insurance trust fund and the Supplementary Medical Insurance trust funds. These funds are in turn financed by the federal government's general fund, payroll taxes, premiums paid by beneficiaries, and out-of-pocket charges. Medicare expenditures in 2023 totaled $839 billion accounting for 14% of total federal spending that year. (30). Why is the source of the funding so important? Because it helps to understand how a tax payer funded government agency has become a haven and treasure chest for private insurers to amass huge fortunes legally. In other words, Medicare Advantage plans have developed legalized scams in the health care industry which are fleecing U.S. taxpayers, physicians, and even worse....patients of quality health care. This will be discussed in more detail in the following chapter.

Chapter 6: The Plot Thickens

As previously mentioned, Medicare Part C was created in 1997 and was dubbed the name Medicare Advantage. This name is only an advantage for the private health insurers behind it. This is another name for the privatized portion of Medicare. Indeed, some reports show that within Medicare Part C Advantage Plans, US tax dollars are funneled through insurance companies so they can take 15% off the top to pay for administrative costs and profit before sending the other 85% to doctors and hospitals who are forced to markedly discount their rates.

Other studies reveal that only 66% of total U.S. healthcare spending goes to medical care. The other 34% goes toward billing, marketing, insurance company profits, and administration. This is in contrast to traditional Medicare which does not transact with insurance companies. Both doctors and hospitals are paid directly by Medicare. Only about 2% of its budget is devoted to administrative costs. Currently, only half of all Medicare beneficiaries are insured by traditional Medicare. Health insurance companies operate as parasites in that they not only survive within Medicare, but they are thriving and at the same time making huge profits. Indeed, reports show that Medicare Advantage Plans make 2.5 times as much profit per enrollee in Medicare as they do from their private sector customers. Even the cost to Medicare Advantage beneficiaries for this insurance is substantially higher than had they remained with traditional Medicare. Recent statistics show that the cost of insuring Medicare beneficiaries through Medicare Advantage Plans was 22%-35% higher representing a difference from $88 billion to instead $144 billion more than it would have been had those beneficiaries remained in traditional Medicare. (31). Despite these huge disparities in cost, Medicare Advantage Plans routinely deny services to tens of thousands of their enrollees every year as well as denying payment or grossly underpaying physicians who provide these services.

Medicare Advantage Plans were intended to give Medicare beneficiaries the choice of access to well-managed care at a lower cost. But something else has happened. Medicare Advantage Plans have monopolized more than 50% of all Medicare. Moreover, they have figured out how to manipulate the Medicare risk codes to establish Medicare Advantage Plans as by far the most profitable branch of large insurance companies. In fact, according to some research, Medicare Advantage will cost Medicare over $600 billion more in the next 8 years than would have been the case if the enrollees had remained in traditional Medicare. (32) Note, that this additional cost is to Medicare, a taxpayer-funded federal government entity. Even though the costs are much greater, most agree that Medicare Advantage enrollees neither receive better care nor do they have better outcomes.

Medicare Advantage plans are essentially private insurance plans that receive funding from both Medicare and their enrollees by payment of monthly premiums. The federal government pays private insurers a fixed amount per month for each patient enrolled in Medicare called a capitated payment. The actual amount depends on the beneficiary's medical records and the expected health care costs in their county. Medicare Advantage plans are a form of "managed care". This means that third-party health insurers have a huge amount of control over the patient's health care. This control is manifested by directing that the patients can only see physicians within their network with exceptions made only if referrals are made by their primary care or another designated physician. Also, the third-party insurer dictates how long and how often the physician can see the patient by restricting compensation only to their fixed limits.

The primary goal of these third-party health insurers is quite distinct from the treating physician who wants to provide the best possible care for the patient. Third-party health insurers aim to spend as little as possible on patient care to maintain their high-profit margin. Another way to achieve that goal is by employing utilization regulations to prevent doctors and hospitals from spending excessively on patient care. This is tightly regulated by the private insurer's requirement of prior authorization which controls physicians' prescriptions for various medications as well as referrals to see subspecialists. (33)

Private health insurers have adopted several legalized scams to maximize their profits. One of these scams is to rigidly deny broad categories or types of claims without taking the time to evaluate whether the specific claim is covered under their plan or policy. In effect, the insurer becomes intentionally oblivious to the facts with the hope that the claim will eventually be dropped. Private health insurers use auditing software, so-called "denial engines", with the intent to lower the amount of money paid to physicians and hospitals.

These auditing programs work by finding technical errors in billing codes required of doctors, hospitals and clinics for submission for payments. These scams not only allow the health insurer to deny payment of claims but also to grossly underpay the claims, if paid. Another scam employed is to make health insurance contracts incredibly complex without stipulating the exact fee schedule that will be paid to doctors. (34). This is a very popular method since the physician has no idea what fee schedule is used for compensation which is typically well below the Medicare rate.

The private health insurer Cigna has built an elaborate system that allows its doctors to instantly reject a claim on medical grounds without opening the patient's file. How is this possible? Reports show that over two months in 2023, Cigna doctors denied over 300,000 claim requests for payments using this method while spending an average of 1.2 seconds on each claim. At the same time, Cigna claims to cover or administer health care plans for 18 million people. In the past, insurance company doctors were required to review claims submitted by doctors before rejecting them on grounds of no medical necessity according to most state laws and regulations. Medical directors are supposed to be designated within insurance companies with the task of examining patient records, reviewing coverage policies, and using their expertise to determine whether it is feasible to approve or deny claims.

However, the Cigna review system completely bypasses this step. Instead, a computer does all the work. Cigna makes use of a computerized algorithm that flags mismatches between diagnoses and what the company considers acceptable tests and procedures for corresponding conditions or infirmities. Company doctors then sign off on the denials in batches without any review. Some Cigna executives questioned whether this procedure was lawful. The idea was shuffled through their legal department and was given the "OK".

Is this a recent practice that Cigna has been using? The painful but simple answer is "no". Cigna adopted its review system more than a decade ago. To make matters even worse, health insurance executives admit that similar systems have previously existed in various forms throughout the industry for some time now. Cigna's denial review system was originally developed by a former pediatrician who reportedly later brought the same computerized algorithm to United Health Care. United Health Care ranks number one in terms of denial of claims for payment by doctors on the grounds of alleged "lack of medical necessity". In contrast, Medicare also has a computerized system that automatically prevents payment of claims by doctors or hospitals that are incorrectly coded. However, Medicare denies payment to doctors on the grounds of lack of medical necessity only when treatments are not considered appropriate or required for a patient's condition based on established medical standards. (35)

It does not require a rocket scientist to understand why private health insurers are making record profits. For example, United Health Care made a record $17.7 billion in profit in 2021. Yet, in 2023, the same United Health Group did even better, raking in $324 billion in revenues behind only giants including Walmart, Amazon, Apple, and Exxon Mobil. They are also the largest private health insurer with 151 million customers representing nearly half of the US population. (36)

Private health insurers have become creative in recent years with several bad-faith tactics with the primary objective of paying as little as possible to doctors and hospitals for their services to patients while amassing huge profits. This also includes payments for the pharmaceutical needs of the patient they claim to provide care for under the auspices of so-called "managed care". Some of these bad faith practices include misrepresentation, which involves providing false information regarding coverage to clients as well as lack of transparency regarding fee schedule payments to doctors in the contracts rendered to them by the private insurer. Insurers go so far as to falsely claim that they have made payments to doctors when they have made no such payments at all. Underpayment is another tactic private health insurers utilize to hold onto profits. The private insurer pays a doctor at a much lower amount than expected or stipulated in their contractual agreement for a given service.

For example, it is generally expected that private health insurers who offer Medicare Advantage plans will compensate a doctor at a higher rate than Medicare. In fact, among five recent studies of primary care services and five studies of specialty services, the Congressional Budget Office found that commercial insurers paid 117% of Medicare Fee For Service rates for primary care services while the same insurers paid 144% of Medicare Fee For Service rates for specialty care services. (37). Another study reported in 2020 revealed that private insurers paid all physicians for their services to patients at an average rate of 143% of Medicare rates, ranging from 118% to 179% of Medicare rates, depending upon the type of doctor and service provided.

The disparity was even greater for hospital services as opposed to clinics or private practices. Private insurers paid for outpatient hospital services at a rate of 264% of Medicare rates while inpatient hospital services were paid at a rate of 189% of Medicare rates. (38) This displays a tendency to favor surgeons and medical subspecialists with significantly higher compensation compared with primary care physicians who primarily practice in a clinic or private practice setting. The trend now is that many commercial health insurers pay primary care doctors well below the Medicare rates which have been steadily decreasing now for more than 20 years. (39)

Another bad faith tactic used by private insurers is a lack of explanation. In other words, the private insurer fails to give a complete or valid justification to a doctor of why the claim has been denied. The most common denial reason is lack of medical necessity. Of note, this determination is frequently made by a computerized algorithm with no physician involvement or review as previously mentioned in the case of Cigna. United Health Care is most notorious for this practice of denying upwards of 33% of their claims to doctors alleging "lack of medical necessity".

Other private insurers will pay part of a claim but refuse to pay for the extra time submitted by the doctor for ancillary procedures performed such as an electrocardiogram done for a patient complaining of chest pain. Private insurers also fail to disclose. This trickery involves not telling a client or stipulating in a contract with a doctor what exactly will be covered with a payment. Furthermore, private insurers prefer to 'bury their heads in the sand' by failing to investigate. They simply refuse to pay a claim without investigating the facts to determine if the claim is justifiable. (40)

There seems to be little, if any, regulation of these bad faith, fraudulent practices by private health insurers. Therefore, a physician has virtually nowhere to go to report a commercial insurer. This is true even though the vast majority of the US population pays for health care by using their health insurance. This problem is especially evident in the case of small primary care clinics or small hospitals, which are extremely vulnerable to behemoth insurance companies. These private health insurers take credit for the physician's care of the patient as well as the huge discounts the physician is forced to concede with the patient visit. Yet, private insurers either simply refuse to pay the doctor for their service, citing no medical necessity, falsely claim to the doctor and/or the patient that they paid for the service provided when they did not. Also, the insurer may grossly underpay the physician at a rate well below the already hugely discounted Medicare rates and deny the extra time submitted in the claim by the doctor or provider for the time spent in caring for the patient. The National Association of Insurance Commissioners supposedly mandates that insurance claims must be handled fairly and that there should be clear communication between both parties.

Nevertheless, insurance companies merely "thumb their nose' at this federal agency because it has no authority nor power to do anything to enforce the law against private insurers. The reason is because states supposedly regulate insurance, not the federal government. (41) But, the truth of the matter is that neither entity, whether state or federal, has the authority to control fraud among insurance companies. Most state insurance commissions have no jurisdiction over many insurance plans and none, whatsoever over Medicare Advantage plans, which are supposedly under the Center for Medicare Services (CMS). Yet, if a physician contacts the Center for Medicare Services regarding the improper or fraudulent conduct of an insurance company, the complaint will likely fall upon deaf ears. Within the Center for Medicare Services, there is no one to call when a health care provider such as a physician is dealt with fraudulently or with bad faith practices by a private insurer who presides over a Medicare Advantage plan. On the other hand, there is a provision to complain if you are a client of the insurance company. The health insurance companies, notoriously known for fraudulent bad faith practices, include United Health Care, Aetna, Cigna, and Anthem.

THE DECIMATION OF U.S. HEALTHCARE

Undoubtedly, as a result of their unscrupulous practices, Medicare Advantage plans have recently come under the spotlight of both the US Department of Justice and the Inspector General. One of the conclusions is that Medicare Advantage plans are significantly overpaid due in part to manipulation of the risk-adjusted payment system used currently. Even though this nefarious manipulation on the part of private insurers is well known by the Center for Medicare Services (CMS), Medicare Advantage plans will annually receive a pay increase. The Center for Medicare Services plans to reward Medicare Advantage plans with an overall pay increase of 3.7% to the tune of $16 billion in 2025!

Who says crime does not pay? The Justice Department has made efforts to pursue cases alleging false claims in the Medicare Advantage plans. For example, the Justice Department has investigated allegations that organizations participating in the program knowingly submitted or caused the submission of inaccurate information or purposely failed to correct information about the health status of beneficiaries enrolled to increase reimbursement. The stakes are extremely high for the US economy since Medicare Advantage plans or Medicare Part C is now the largest component of Medicare both in terms of federal dollars spent and the number of beneficiaries.

The Department of Justice has reached settlements for this fraudulent behavior with giants like Cigna and Martin Point. The Department of Justice has ongoing litigation against corporate giants like United Health Group, Independent Health Corporation, Elevance Health, and Kaiser Permanente for the same behavior. United Health Group is by far the largest Medicare Advantage insurer in the US. It seems that the Medicare Advantage plan model relies on providing as little care as possible in general.

At the same time, insurers put care approval behind a wall of delays and denials to save money and leave patients suffering without necessary treatment. (42)

Since the private health insurers have closely mimicked the Physician Fee Schedule of Medicare over the years, the stage has been set for a growing fiscal crisis for the recipients of both, namely US physicians. It must be kept in mind that Medicare is a federal government agency primarily funded by payroll taxes which comes from US taxpayers. Because it is a federal agency, it has a fixed budget that must be balanced annually. Regarding hospitals, Medicare adopted its prospective payment system in 1983. This system sets payment rates for hospitals in advance based on categories of service known as Diagnosis Related Groups (DRGs).

Congress created the Sustainable Growth Rate (SGR) to account for rising hospital and practice costs as a result of advancing technology, cost of living increases, and increases in inflation. In the beginning, the SGR had to be repeatedly modified and factored into Medicare payments to physicians and hospitals to prevent annual reductions in Medicare payments. However, as with many well-intentioned ideas, it was ultimately repealed by lawmakers. This left doctors and hospitals without any protection against future Medicare payment cuts that would fail to keep pace with rapidly increasing practice costs. The fear was that as a result of no longer factoring in SGRs into Medicare payments, hospitals and physician practices would be rendered fiscally unsustainable, ultimately jeopardizing patient care. (43).

This has indeed become a self-fulfilling prophecy. Medicare physician payments declined an astounding 29% from 2001 to 2024. This has occurred despite 2023 being dubbed as the year with the highest inflation rate in more than 40 years! It is obvious that Medicare physician payments neither take into account trending economic conditions, rising inflation nor rising practice costs due to advances in science and technology as well as cost of living increases. In 2024 alone, practice cost inflation increases will be 3.6% higher. The Medicare physician payment reduction is gradually increasing in recent years. For example, Medicare reduced payments to physicians in 2023 by 2%. In 2024, Medicare cut the rate to physicians by an additional 1.69%. Congress has recently approved an additional Medicare payment reduction to physicians in 2025 of a shocking 2.8%!.(44).

To make matters worse, private health insurers have been allowed to charge doctors from 1.5% to 5% with each payment electronically directly deposited in their account. The Center for Medicare Services (CMS) originally prohibited fees for electronic funds transfers until this prohibition was successfully lobbied by the payment processor, Zelis. This caused CMS to change its position in 2018 and to reverse course completely in 2022 stating that such fees are not prohibited, There is currently bipartisan legislation that may prohibit this practice by private health insurers, which adds up to billions of dollars. (45). Not to mention the fact that most electronic health records are financially linked to a third-party billing merchant who charges more than 3% for every transaction made with the swipe of a credit card in their respective offices. This is another example of the legalized fleecing of physicians by third-party health insurers and corporate entities.

Private health insurers have also been steadily decreasing payments to physicians over the past 20 years due to fee schedules that are purposely developed to closely mimic Medicare rates. Yet, health insurance annual premiums continue to rise. For example, the average annual health insurance premium in 2023 was $8,435 for single coverage and $23,968 for family coverage. The average annual premium for both single coverage and family coverage has risen by 22% just since 2018. (46) The median proposed increase in 2024 was 6%, ranging from 2%-10% nationwide. Ironically, the justification for the rate increases was primarily the increase in the cost of health care. Specific reasons given included an increase in the "unit" cost of services primarily from hospitals, physicians, and pharmaceutical companies.

Other reasons given for the increase in premiums included inflation and the COVID-19 pandemic. According to private insurers, inflation is in part responsible for a rise in premiums due to growth in prices paid by insurers for medical services and medications, as well as growth in the utilization of health care. (47). Strangely enough, these are all factors cited by physicians as to why their payments should be increased. However, this same justification used by private insurers for increasing premiums has fallen on deaf ears in Congress when used by physicians to request higher reimbursement from Medicare and by extension, from the private insurers. The current trend is heading for a perfect storm, a fiscal catastrophe of monumental proportions for physicians. This is especially true for so-called primary care physicians. Furthermore, doom and gloom are what the near future forecasts for primary care doctors who choose to have a solo practice or to practice in a small group. The same is true for small hospitals. These issues will be discussed further in the next chapter.

Chapter 7: Primary Care Physicians, Small Hospitals and Clinics: How the Backbone Was Broken

Primary care has been notoriously categorized by private insurers for simplification of payment much to the demise of the US health care system, not to mention the tremendous financial harm to physicians. Primary care providers include physician assistants, nurse practitioners who are trained in family practice, General practitioners who have completed medical school and one year of Internship and Residency, Family Practice physicians, who have completed medical school along with a three-year Residency in Family Practice, Pediatricians, who have completed medical school with a three-year Residency in the specialty of Pediatrics (which involves the medical care of infants, children, and adolescents) and finally, Internal Medicine physicians, who complete medical school and a three-year Residency in the specialty of Internal Medicine (which involves the medical care of adults and includes adolescents).

These vastly different professions are placed by private health insurers in the same payment category It is obvious that these providers have dramatically different education and levels of training. Yet, they are all compensated at the same rate by Medicare and by private insurers. Indeed, the specialties of Pediatrics and Internal Medicine are not even considered specialists according to the categories of the private insurers. They are simply lumped together as primary care providers. Not only is this 'lump sum' category demeaning, but it also puts those labeled within it in fiscal peril. Medicare and private health insurers utilize this same system for reimbursement purposes by assigning 'providers' as 'primary care provider' (PCP) or 'specialist'.

However, this system is deeply problematic. Why? Consider this: Medicare covers people 65 years of age and over along with those who have certain disabilities. This accounts for approximately 65 million people in the US encompassing more than a fifth of all health care spending nationwide. Furthermore, those who primarily take care of these people, most with chronic disease, are primary care providers. Chief among them are mainly Internal Medicine doctors who care for adolescents and adults and Pediatricians who care for infants and children. These two groups also provide the bulk of the hospital-based care as hospitalists due to their uniquely suited training to care for chronic and acute diseases in these two populations' settings.

Yet, Medicare has been decreasing its physician payment rates for over 20 consecutive years. To make matters worse, Medicare has traditionally placed a much greater value on surgery and medical procedures versus the methodical clinical acumen needed to make an accurate diagnosis and administer the appropriate treatment. For this reason, there exists a widening disparity in reimbursement for primary care providers versus surgical subspecialties who perform surgery or medical subspecialists who perform medical procedures. The private insurers do the same, basing their payment amounts on the Medicare system. A primary care physician, especially Internal Medicine, may have to spend hours of unreimbursed time evaluating a patient.

This may include meticulous history taking, performing a detailed physical exam, and reviewing previous medical records, labs, and imaging studies to arrive at a correct diagnosis and to prescribe the best treatment for the patient. Also, the patient's care may involve phone calls or referrals to other sub-specialists, phone calls with the patient, responding to e-mails from the patient, reviewing new labs or imaging studies, as well as consultation reports and informing the patient either in writing or by phone, refilling prescription requests or filling out legal forms that the patient may need. All of these things consume much time but are not compensated for by Medicare or by private health insurers.

Medicare has at times, attempted to level the playing field somewhat by introducing various codes which allow greater reimbursement for primary care providers. Yet, Medicare is advised by the American Medical Association (AMA) annually regarding its budget, which is fixed. Unfortunately, the balance of power is leveraged against primary care providers (PCPs). The American College of Surgeons, along with 18 other medical subspecialty groups all within the AMA, routinely oppose the implementation of any new billing codes for complex patient evaluation and management services.

These are services unique to the specialty of Internal Medicine in the care of adults and to the specialty of Pediatrics in the care of infants and children. The reason is that these codes would increase reimbursement to primary care providers while simultaneously decreasing reimbursement to surgeons and medical subspecialists since Medicare operates on a fixed annual budget. (48). Many private insurers either refuse to pay these billing codes which represent extra time spent with the patient or will only pay a limited amount. In most cases, the payment is far short of what the doctor submits as the time spent with the patient and the payment rate is extremely low. It is easy to see why primary care physicians are unable to sustain their practices—the only way to maintain a survivable income in this environment is to markedly increase your patient volume, which means seeing a lot of patients a day in an ultra-rushed fashion.

Primary care is unique in that it is the only part of the US health system in which the services result in better population health and better health outcomes. Without primary care, minor health problems can easily spiral into a chronic or terminal disease. The results without primary care will be poor disease management and emergency room overuse along with unsustainable costs. A recent study showed that US adults who regularly see a primary care physician have 33% lower healthcare costs and a 19% lower risk of dying prematurely than those who see only a subspecialist. Yet, US healthcare largely functions by sending patients from one specialist to another for problems that could easily be cared for by a good Internal Medicine physician. Furthermore, it has been shown that the US could save up to $67 billion a year if everyone used a primary care physician as their principal source of care.

This translates into $13 in savings for every $1 increase in primary care spending! The sensible and logical thing to do is for everyone to have a primary care physician. But the facts show quite the opposite.

Primary care physicians are on life support in the US and are becoming virtually extinct. Why? The problem with reimbursement has already been discussed. Most primary care physician's income is based upon either highly unreliable or low-paying sources. The reason is that most people want to pay for their care at office visits by using their commercial insurance or Medicare or Medicaid. The majority of physicians have no other option but to accept the markedly discounted rates of reimbursement by the latter two federal government entities which are generally reliable about payments. Yet, commercial health insurance companies reimburse physicians at a markedly discounted rate, many times even below the Medicare rate. To make matters worse, commercial insurance companies routinely deny payments to physicians without justification or consequences.

This is especially true with primary care physicians in small clinics as opposed to large groups of physicians who usually have access to billing departments to ensure payment. This also applies to small hospitals. As is the case in any business, without a steady robust income, a primary care practice cannot survive. Largely due to this problem, primary care physicians are leaving the practice of medicine in droves. Thus, there is a growing shortage of primary care physicians in the U.S.

The COVID-19 pandemic truly exposed a tremendous weakness in the US healthcare system. Primary care physicians, who represent the backbone of US health care were at the forefront during the pandemic and unfortunately, were many of the first to die or to become hospitalized. This left an even greater shortage of primary care physicians, causing those remaining to have to see a greater number of patients regularly. There is also a need for those physicians remaining to face the administrative burden brought about by third-party health insurers' requirements. As a result, a cycle of physician burnout became rampant. This led to a massive exodus of primary care physicians, either in the form of early retirement or transitioning to other forms of practice. One of these alternatives is concierge practices. These practices allow the physician to significantly reduce the volume of patients seen daily and to devote more time to individual patient care. Other physicians have chosen to switch entirely to another method of making a living. Due to this perfect storm of low income and rising medical school debt, a rapidly dwindling number of medical students are going into primary care. The fact is that subspecialty medicine or surgery offers a much more lucrative future than primary care which is hard to ignore. This means that the US will face a projected crippling shortage of 21,000 to 55,000 primary care physicians by 2033 according to the AMA.(49)

What is igniting this massive physician burnout and how widespread is the problem? Studies show that burnout does not only encompass practicing physicians but also extends to residents in training as physicians and even to medical students. A recent survey revealed that 60% of physicians and residents and 70% of medical students reported burnout while this figure was only at 40% before the COVID-19 pandemic. This burnout has led to a markedly higher suicide rate among this group. A great contributing factor includes stresses engendered by changes in the healthcare environment as a result of acquisitions and mergers brought about by private equity takeover of the health care industry. As a result of these mergers and acquisitions by private equity, 50% of those surveyed reported negative job satisfaction, 36% reported that this caused a lower quality of patient care, 30% felt that it raised patient health care costs and 35% agreed that independent medical judgment was negatively impacted. Furthermore, 70% of the physicians and medical students surveyed felt that consolidation by these means was adversely affecting patient access to high-quality and cost-efficient care.

Also, mergers and acquisitions of healthcare institutions by private equity have left physicians feeling as though they have lost the autonomy they once had, which also contributes greatly to burnout. The reason for this is that under the oversight of so-called "managed care" by private health insurers and private equity opportunists, a physician is no longer able to make medical decisions that are in the patient's best interest. Even though the physician is ultimately held responsible for whatever happens to the patient, they do not have complete control over patient outcomes, which contributes to burnout. Interestingly, 40% of those surveyed were primary care physicians while 60% were specialists. Most (75%) were employed physicians and 50% were 45 years of age or younger. (50)

This highlights another dramatic change in health care in the US. From 2012 to 2022, the number of physicians who work in private practice decreased by 13% from 60.1% to 46.7%. Yet, these numbers include not only physicians who own the practice but also physician employees of the practice. Over that same 10-year period, physicians directly employed by or who contracted directly with a hospital increased from 5.6% to 9.6%. The vast majority of hospitalists, physicians who solely take care of patients during their hospitalization, are Internal Medicine physicians, which is a rapidly growing field. Also, those who worked in a hospital-owned practice increased from 23.4% to 31.3%.

The overwhelming reason cited by 80% of physicians as to why they were forced to sell their practice to a hospital or a private equity health care system was the need to negotiate higher payment rates with third-party payers (private health insurers). (51). Notably, private health insurer's burdensome regulatory and administrative requirements were given by 71% of those surveyed as the second biggest reason for selling their practices. The third greatest reason given by 69% of those surveyed to sell their practice was the failure to improve access to costly resources. (52) It seems that the main reasons for the trend from solo practice to direct or indirect hospital employment is a combination of factors including mandatory annual payment cuts to Medicare which private health insurers mimic, steadily rising practice costs, and burdensome and often unrelenting regulations and restrictions on payment imposed by private health insurers. The effect of this shift has been monumental for primary care physicians. Among physicians in hospital-owned practices, 61% were affiliated with practices that include primary care compared to 44.9% of those in private practice. The trend is away from small practices and toward larger practices.

Corporate giants are gradually taking over the healthcare industry. Even insurance companies have joined in the takeover by purchasing clinics. (53). For example, CVS Health recently bought Oak Street's fast-growing chain of primary care centers that employ doctors in 21 states of the US (54). Currently, some of the nation's largest health insurers are opening their primary care clinics. This move allows them to control both the payment and delivery of care. Both CVS and Aetna are expanding with Minute Clinics that boast no co-pay for members. United Health Care offers a health plan in Los Angeles that is based upon their Optum physicians, surgery centers and urgent-care clinics in the area. Blue Cross & Blue Shield of Houston and Dallas, Texas offer its members free primary care visits at specific clinics in those respective areas. Kaiser Permanente already owns its network of hospitals and doctors. Even Humana has partnered with a private equity firm to expand primary care delivery to its Medicare members as well as to take hold of home health involving visiting nurses and the hospice sectors. (55)

Private equity takeovers of the US health system have had a devastating effect on communities. Large hospital systems are closing their locations in lower-income communities. The effect of these closures leaves individuals faced with the choice of whether or not to seek medical care and if so, to be burdened with overwhelming debt. Private equity takeovers of the healthcare industry have proven to be very profitable for giant corporations. In fact, in 2021 alone, there were 1400 private equity deals in health care amounting to $209 billion. Moreover, there has been a sixfold increase in the number of physician offices acquired by private equity over the last ten years. The takeover has extended to hospitals with 30% of for-profit hospitals now owned by private equity. A prevailing result of private equity acquisition has been much higher healthcare costs and increases in patient mortality. (56)

This trend toward private equity consolidation has obligated physicians to become employees of nonphysician healthcare corporations. The result has been very detrimental to both the physician and the patient as well as to the US economy. Private equity mergers and acquisitions of healthcare systems have not only resulted in a monopoly of consumer choice but also increased healthcare costs due to monopolizing the physician workforce. Corporate greed dominating US health care has resulted in anti-competitive labor practices that lead to intimidation of and retaliation against physicians who advocate for patients.

It has also led to corporations increasingly replacing physicians with lesser-trained non-physician practitioners such as nurse practitioners and physician assistants of whom less compensation is exacted. For example, a nurse practitioner obtains a 4-year degree in Nursing and then completes a Masters or Doctor of Nursing which takes anywhere from 18 months to 3 years to complete. On the other hand, a physician assistant completes a 4-year degree and goes on to complete a 2-year Master's Degree as a physician assistant. Compare this to the average physician who completes a 4-year undergraduate degree usually in Premedical studies, graduates from a

4-year Medical School, and then completes at least at least a 1-year internship/residency.

However, most physicians complete at least a 3-year internship/residency. Many physicians go on to complete fellowship training to become medical sub-specialists or surgeons. By replacing physicians with nonphysician practitioners, private equity can falsely portray these practitioners as real physicians while paying them significantly less. In this way, large corporations can maximize their profits while increasing costs to patients and taxpayers. More importantly, the quality of health care is dramatically lowered without the real physician's expertise and experience to manage a patient correctly. (57). This is even much more the case as patients are presenting sicker than ever with more complexities as time moves on. The latter is especially true in the United States.

Private equity has now gone after emergency rooms across the U.S. in addition to hospitals. Since aiming its attention at the current 4.8 trillion dollars healthcare industry, private equity has come a long way since its beginning in the late 1980s. Corporate giant takeovers in health care began around 2000 and since that time have steadily increased now, even expanding to 25% of emergency rooms in the U.S.

How have they accomplished this? For many years, physician staffing in many emergency rooms in the U.S. was operated by coop-like groups under the direction of working doctors who contracted with hospitals. But in the 1990s, former physicians and other enterprises began taking ownership of contract management groups (CMGs). This initiated the process of these entities acting like profit-making businesses, centralizing decision-making and earnings. So private equity began to take over CMGs acquiring more and more emergency rooms. In fact, by 2009, almost 9% of ER doctor groups were owned by private equity. By 2019, the number jumped to 22%. As of March 2024, 25% of ER doctor groups in the U.S. are owned by private equity. However, when private corporations buy out these CMGs, they are not purchasing along with the CMGs, buildings, staff, land, or medical equipment. What they are purchasing is ownership of the board-certified emergency physicians in exchange for huge payouts to physician owners of the CMGs. In other words, they are uniquely acquiring the expertise and services of the physicians in exchange for a price. Hospitals for-profit prefer private equity ownership over doctor-owned CMGs. Why? The simple answer is that they make a lot more money. Private equity that takes over an ER can profit in one or both of two ways: The corporate interest can maximize what it charges for patient services or it can cut what it pays to clinicians who provide those services.

What have been the results of these acquisitions by private equity? Just as firms pressure their employees to take care of the customer as fast as possible to maximize revenue, private equity pressures clinicians to see patients as fast as possible. Many even impose penalties on the physician if the patient is not seen within 25 minutes of arriving at the ER. At times, this may be a tall order in a busy ER with patients coming in at a rapid pace, some in critical condition. For example, patients with stab or gunshot wounds, patients involved in motor vehicle accidents, medical emergencies like a heart attack or stroke, or surgical emergencies such as a ruptured aortic aneurysm, may arrive all at once. This has resulted in dangerously rushed decision-making. In some cases, this type of rushed care has compromised otherwise delivery of good patient care by the physician. Firms also pressure physicians to recommend admission to the hospital for most patients, even if this is medically unnecessary. Private equity has also dramatically raised prices for many emergency services which has led to astronomical bills to patients for emergency room services.

In addition, private equity entities recognize that it is much easier to collect from individual patients than from insurance companies that have computerized programs aimed at denying payment. Therefore, firms have restricted participation in insurance networks knowing that patients must pay if the service received is not covered by insurance. As a result, costs to patients have skyrocketed. One study revealed that costs went up more than 80% as a result of corporate interest's takeover of an ER and a hospital. Another way private equity has minimized their costs and overhead is by replacing more expensive physicians with nurse practitioners and physician assistants as previously discussed There is no question that this move has significantly lowered the quality of health care rendered and has no doubt worsened patient outcomes. (58)

Corporate takeovers of emergency rooms have dramatically adversely affected emergency physicians financially. For example, NES Health, a physician staffing company, recently sent out an ominous e-mail to its emergency physicians. The physicians were informed that NES Health did not have enough money to pay them this month. The message explained that due to "necessary operational transitions", the company experienced a "temporary shortfall in monthly revenue". A loan for this purpose could not be obtained. Furthermore, the company did not explain how long it would take to pay the amount owed. Physicians were left worried about the financial stability of the company they worked for. Many were concerned that this would be as was the case with American Physician Practices, who filed for bankruptcy in 2023 and shortly thereafter, Envision who did the same. Both are physician staffing companies. NES Health staffs 35 emergency departments in the U.S. The largest physician staffing companies in the country are Team Health and U.S. Acute Care Solutions, which staff 562 and 101 emergency departments in the nation, respectively. Although the exact ownership of NES Health is unclear, this situation has raised serious concerns among physicians regarding private equity firms having ownership of physician staffing companies. (59)

Medicare Advantage plans have also greatly contributed to the decimation of the US healthcare system inflicting economic blows not only to physicians, especially primary care physicians, but also to taxpayers. Medicare Advantage was created by Congress in 2003 under the Medicare Modernization Act. Ironically, the purpose was to help stabilize healthcare spending on the elderly. But instead, these plans have dramatically driven up healthcare costs nationwide. Medicare Advantage plans, backed by private commercial insurers, cover nearly 16 million Americans at a cost of more than $150 billion in 2024. These plans are very popular. Why? The claim is that the plans fill the gaps in coverage, with less out-of-pocket expense, and offer extra benefits including dental and eye care.

Yet, billions of dollars are misspent every year through so-called billing errors linked to a payment tool called a "risk score". Medicare uses a formula to calculate this risk score which has led to gross abuse and fraud by Medicare Advantage plans. Supposedly, Medicare Advantage plans are paid higher rates for sicker patients with a higher risk score and lower amounts for healthier patients with a lower risk score. As previously mentioned, a monthly payment is paid by Medicare to these Medicare Advantage plans in the form of a capitated payment varying according to the county a person resides. However, shrewd individuals behind Medicare

Advantage plans have found ways to manipulate these risk scores, much to their financial advantage. For example, from 2008 to 2013, risk scores shuffled nearly $70 billion in "improper" payments to Medicare Advantage plans into the coffers of private health insurers. Risk scores of Medicare Advantage plans rose exponentially in 1000 counties nationwide from 2007 to 2011. This sharp rise resulted in taxpayer spending of more than $36 billion over estimated costs for patients in standard Medicare. Furthermore, in more than 200 of those counties, the cost of some Medicare Advantage plans were at least 25% higher than the cost of providing traditional Medicare. (60)

Congress detected the abuse of these Medicare Advantage plans in 2005. To rein in costs, CMS was directed to include an annual coding intensity adjustment to reduce Medicare Advantage risk scores to be more in line with traditional Medicare. However, since 2018, CMS has only been able to set the "coding adjustment" at 5.9% which is the minimum amount required by law. Medicare Advantage plans continue to find new and creative ways to increase their enrollee's risk scores, which translates into higher monthly payments from Medicare. Attempts to reduce capitated payments from Medicare-to-Medicare Advantage plans have been met with vehement opposition by lawmakers, including Senators. The financial burden of this fraud has long been passed on to taxpayers, who pay much more for Medicare Advantage plan enrollees than those enrolled in traditional Medicare. (61)

Most of us probably feel that it would be easy to investigate and punish those participating in this massive fraud and abuse. Nevertheless, it has been virtually impossible for the federal government to trace hundreds of millions of dollars lost in suspected overpayments to Medicare Advantage plans that date back as far as 2007.

In fact, the Affordable Care Act (Obama Care), mandated significant rate cuts to capitated payments given to Medicare Advantage plans in part, to cover millions of uninsured people. Nevertheless, this initiative was met with stiff opposition by Medicare Advantage plan lobbyists backed by private health insurers. These third-party insurers quickly enlisted the support and help of Congress. As a result, the rate cuts to Medicare Advantage plans were stopped. Thus, while health insurance premiums with Medicare Advantage plans continue to rise annually, the taxpayer-funded capitated payments to these plans have not been cut, and in fact, are rising. The Center for Public Integrity found that Medicare Advantage plans can cost the federal government as much as 25% more than traditional Medicare. (62)

Also, the Affordable Care Act, passed by Congress in 2010 with key provisions beginning January 1, 2014, has been great news for private health insurers. With lofty goals to expand health care for millions of low-income people and to eliminate denial of coverage on the grounds of pre-existing conditions, the ACA has resulted in big profits for health insurance companies. Despite significant financial losses in the individual market after the key provisions of the ACA took effect, health insurers' profitability in the individual market has risen substantially. This profit windfall is largely due to significant premium increases, government premium tax credits that pay for those premium increases, and the large government-funded Medicaid expansion. It seems that insurers who remained in the individual and small group markets have acquired an older and more costly risk pool than expected which has allowed them under ACA regulations to charge much higher premiums. These premiums have largely been funded by taxpayer-generated federal government subsidies.

The stable year-to-year enrollment, despite large premium increases, suggests a distorted market that involves large transfers from taxpayers to third-party health insurers. Many of the larger insurance companies who left the individual market are profiting from the Medicaid expansion, primarily provided through private "managed care" and paid for by the federal government. Approximately 85% of exchange purchases receive a premium subsidy. These subsidies are computed so that enrollees do not pay more than a prescribed portion of their income for a common plan. This ensures that insurance companies will receive subsidies regardless of how high the premiums go which reduces incentives for price competition as taxpayers fund almost all of the higher premiums. (63)

In fiscal year 2023, federal subsidies through the ACA Medicaid expansion and exchanges have cost the federal government $218 billion with practically all of the money going to private health insurers and not to physicians, who provide the health care. About half of all U.S. healthcare spending amounting to $4.8 trillion in 2023 and the majority of private health insurer revenue now comes directly from the taxpayer-funded federal government. Unfortunately, the ACA has led to inflationary premiums and spending often with little to no value to patients along with even greater reliance on the government. As a result, the private health insurer stock prices have gone through the roof, up an astronomical 1032% since 2010 when the ACA was enacted. The stocks have surged 448% since 2013, the year before the implementation of its key provisions.

The ACAs Medicaid expansion has produced even greater profits for private health insurers. Federal spending on expansion enrollees was $126 billion in 2023. The state share would add another $13 billion contribution to private health insurer's treasure chests. Using inflation-adjusted dollars for comparison, Medicaid spending with payments to private health insurers nearly quadrupled from 2010 to 2021. Insurers have also benefited from loose state eligibility determinations that have allowed millions of people to be placed in a Medicaid managed care plan who are not eligible or without proper eligibility reviews.

Furthermore, the ACA transformed the unsubsidized individual market into a market with much higher premiums that people typically need massive subsidies to afford. These subsidies give private insurers significant leverage to increase premium prices as the burden of any additional expense is almost entirely borne by taxpayers. The Congressional Budget Office estimates that these subsidies equaled $92 billion in 2023. President Biden signed legislation that significantly expanded these subsidies, essentially making zero-premium plans available to many enrollees. Ironically, this legislation originally targeting a lower-income population, has made these subsidies available to some with household incomes among the top 5% in the U.S. (64)

The pharmaceutical industry is another private sector of the healthcare industry that has benefitted greatly from federal government policies even though this sector has been allowed to dramatically raise drug prices for patients. For example, in 2018, Americans spent $535 billion on prescription drugs. This represented an increase of 50% since 2010. From 2011 to 2015 alone the prices of prescription drugs increased anywhere from 40% to 71%. A study found that the price of Insulin doubled from

2012 to 2018. In the ten years from 2002 to 2012, the price of Insulin nearly tripled. Yet, despite these massive price increases passed on to consumers, a 2018 report showed that $100 billion funded by taxpayers went to the National Institute of Health (NIH) for research and development of 210 drugs approved by the Food and Drug Administration (FDA) from 2010 to 2016.

Since 1981, pharmaceutical companies have also benefited from substantial tax credits for research and development. In fact, in 2015, then-President Barack Obama signed into law the Protecting Americans from Tax Hike which made these tax credits permanent and even extended this provision to small businesses and startup companies. Furthermore, the pharmaceutical industry receives tax deductions for their marketing and advertising expenses which include television commercials and social media. Not to mention, a corporate tax cut of 14% allowed pharmaceutical companies in 2018 to pocket $76 billion! However, despite these huge taxpayer-funded subsidies issued by the federal government, in 2019 drug manufacturers still raised prices on more than 3,400 drugs. (65)

While the healthcare industry has become gradually dominated by big business and corporate greed, a more subtle attack has been developing. But this attack is against the principal component of any health care system, the physician. It seems that the attacks have been spearheaded by the U.S. government. As far back as the 1970s, the Rural Health Care Act of 1977 was enacted to replace physicians. This law mandated that to receive federal funding, no less than 50% of all services had to be provided by a nurse practitioner or a physician assistant. In the 1980s, the federal government enacted policies to restrict physician growth. For example, in 1997 a cap was placed on funding for residency training programs, even though all medical school graduates are required to complete at least one year of residency to become licensed physicians in the U.S. Despite alarm warnings of a looming physician shortage, bills presented to reverse the freeze on funding of residency training have failed to pass in Congress almost every year since 2007.

The federal government has promoted policies to worsen the physician shortage. How? By reducing the number of physician graduates while promoting the number of nurse practitioners and physician assistants. President Bill Clinton pushed legislation for $200 million to be allocated to fund nurse practitioner training. Fifteen years later, in 2010, then President Barack Obama signed the Affordable Care Act which expanded funding to both nurse practitioners and physician assistants training programs without increasing funding for residency training for physicians. In 2016, the Veteran's Administration began to allow nurse practitioners to occupy the role previously held by physicians which allowed them to treat servicemen and women independently without physician supervision. In 2019, the U.S. Government Accountability Office went so far as to recommend diverting physician residency training funding toward spending only for nurse practitioner and physician assistant so-called 'residency' programs. Even the recent Biden administration allocated $100 million specifically to train nurse practitioners how to own and operate primary care practices.

Are these efforts to replace physicians with non-physicians working? The short answer is "no". Nurse practitioners enhance and complement physicians, but do not replace them. This is due to major differences in education, training, and scope of practice. For these reasons, complex cases and specialized care are best handled by a physician. ((66),(67). Also, nurse practitioners and physician assistants are leaving primary care for the same reasons physicians are leaving: poor pay and burnout. The reality is that only 30% of physicians and 33% of physician assistants choose primary care. Only 48% of nurse practitioners worked in primary care in 2012. Yet, even after a $179 million federally funded pilot project was launched in 2019 purposed to encourage nurse practitioners to choose primary care, the effort dismally failed. Currently, in 2024 only 12% of nurse practitioner program graduates entered the field of primary care.

Why are so many leaving primary care? Patients are coming in sicker and with more complexities than ever before. Yet, clinicians are being asked to evaluate them in a brief period and at the same time maintain high patient satisfaction. They also have to deal with the administrative burden of third-party insurers which can take hours, especially when managed care and authorizations are involved. Studies show that for every 1 hour spent by a physician in direct patient care, 2 hours are spent in computer documentation. Not to mention, time spent reviewing labs, charts, answering e-mails, phone calls, and other correspondence from either patients or from referral subspecialists involved in the patient's care which largely goes uncompensated.

A 2022 report by the Hattiesburg Clinic, one of the largest accountable care organizations in the U.S. found that despite caring for panels of lower-risk patients, nurse practitioners and physician assistants working independently had poorer outcomes and higher costs of care than primary care physicians. Physicians were found to perform better in 9 out of 10 quality measures, Moreover, nonphysician practitioners had higher emergency room referrals and specialty referrals costing more than $28.5 million annually. The quality of health care is vitally important and is waning in this country due to those who make policies. The facts reveal that more people die worldwide due to poor quality care than to lack of access to any care at all.

The evidence is clear that primary care physicians are essential for the health care system to remain viable due to interventions that reduce morbidity and mortality. For example, this is accomplished by routine management of risk factors for cardiovascular disease that can lead to death from heart attacks, strokes, and peripheral vascular disease. Measures employed include dietary recommendations and medication to control blood pressure, cholesterol, and Diabetes. Also, primary care physicians can reduce mortality by performing evidence-based screening tests to detect and treat cancer in the earliest stages. There is no doubt that when a person sees a physician over time who has gotten the chance to know them, there is a significant reduction in mortality. The benefits of continuity of care cannot be overstated. This is in part because the physician is trained to perform these services with each visit even when a patient presents with a minor problem. (68). However, most health insurance companies strive to have patients switch their plans which means a different healthcare provider or physician every year!

Yet, the irony of all these facts is that the very providers of medical care, primarily physicians, and especially primary care physicians, have faced Medicare cuts annually for 23 consecutive years amounting to an astonishing 29% rate cut. Even worse, physicians face another 2.8% cut in payments by Medicare beginning January 1, 2025. All private health insurers, including those backing Medicare Advantage plans, will also decrease correspondingly their payment rates to physicians. All this is occurring while practice costs continue to rise, medical education has become exorbitantly expensive, inflation is near an all-time high, and the cost of living has dramatically increased. So, where do we go from here? What can be done to fix the broken healthcare system that is being decimated from within and dominated from without? These questions will be answered in the next chapter.

Chapter 8: A Failing Health Care System: Is There Any Hope for A Revival?

The verdict is in: The US Health Care System is failing. As previously mentioned, much of US health care is dominated by so-called "managed care". This is another name for private health insurers or private equity corporations that operate networks of hospitals and clinics. What are the results? Managed care has left people either with no other option but to change doctors, not to be permitted to go to the doctor they wanted to see, or to be denied needed medical procedures or surgery. To make matters worse, most health insurance plans require patients to change the plan and usually, the doctor every year.

This is because no doctor is credentialed in every single insurance plan by a given health insurance company. This results in the opposite of promoting good quality health care since patients are left almost annually with a new doctor who knows little to nothing about their health history. In contrast, good quality health care can be achieved by continuity of care which means having the same physician for years. This type of care has also resulted in higher healthcare costs and poorer healthcare outcomes. Managed care-controlled employer health care policies have come to favor the employer rather than the employee as the customer they want to please. (69). Even so, these employer health policies are immensely popular, primarily due to the tax reduction incentive attached to offering and receiving them.

There is an old saying: "You get what you pay for". Yet, this seems to be the opposite with regard to US health care. The dismal facts show that while the US spends far more on health care than any other high-income country in the world, the US has the worst health care outcomes overall of any other highly developed country. For example, in 2022, the U.S. spent 17.3 % of their gross domestic product (GDP), a total of $4.5 trillion, on health care which was nearly twice as much as the average highly developed country. This amounts to $13,493 per person in the U.S. This means that health care spending per person in the U.S. was almost twice as much as in the second-highest country which was Germany, and four times higher than in South Korea.

In the U.S., this includes spending for those enrolled in programs including Medicaid, the Children's Health Insurance Program, Medicare, and military plans as well as spending by those with private employer-sponsored coverage or other private insurance and out-of-pocket health care spending. Yet, with all this spending, Americans are more likely to die younger and from avoidable causes than those living in similarly highly developed countries. Indeed, the U.S. has the lowest life expectancy at birth, the highest death rates for avoidable or treatable conditions, the highest maternal and infant mortality, and has among the highest suicide rates So the report card is far from good.

Chronic care management is sorely lacking in the U.S. healthcare system. The U.S. has the highest rate of people with multiple chronic conditions and an obesity rate nearly twice the Organization for Economic Co-operation and Development (OECD) average. Americans also see physicians less often than people in most other high-income countries averaging only 4 visits per year. Despite the highest healthcare spending in the world, the U.S. has the lowest rate of practicing physicians and hospital beds per 1,000 population. This well below-average supply of physicians compared to other OECD countries may in part be the reason for the less frequent physician visits. This is likely especially true in rural or remote areas of the U.S. The average hospital stay of 4.8 days is much lower than in other OECD countries. One bright spot in U.S. health care was cancer screening for breast and colorectal cancer as well as high Influenza vaccination rates. However, COVID-19 vaccination rates lag far behind many developed nations. The sad irony is that since the beginning of the COVID-19 pandemic, more have died from Coronavirus in the U.S. than in any other highly developed country. Indeed, it is estimated that for every 1 million cases of COVID-19 between 1/22/2020 to 1/18/2025, there were more than 3000 deaths in the U.S.

The Inflation Reduction Act will likely help to reduce the high cost of certain drugs including Insulin and to put limits on out-of-pocket expenses, especially for elderly and debilitated ones on Medicare. However, the report concluded that there is a dire need to reduce healthcare and administrative costs to downsize U.S. healthcare spending. The vast majority of the administrative costs come from private health insurers and private equity which dominate health care in the U.S. currently. Another factor of critical importance cited was the need for better prevention and management of chronic diseases. The report highlighted the need to develop the capacity to offer comprehensive, continuous, well-coordinated care. The authors noted that the U.S. has gone for decades underinvesting in effective primary care programs. Furthermore, the U.S. has an inadequate supply of primary care providers. Both of these major factors have limited many in the U.S.'s access to effective primary care, which is the backbone of any healthcare system.

The analysis emphasized the critical requirements of a successful healthcare system. It is essential that the health care system supports chronic disease prevention and management. It is necessary for a health care system to promote early diagnosis and treatment of medical problems. A viable health care system should have affordable access to health care coverage. Finally, a healthcare system should have effective cost-containment measures. (70)

Focusing a spotlight on this OECD data has shed some alarming details regarding the state of U.S. healthcare. For example, despite spending almost twice as much per capita on health care compared to similarly large and wealthy nations, the U.S. has a lower life expectancy than peer nations and has seen worsening measures of health outcomes since the COVID-19 pandemic. Although the COVID-19 pandemic resulted in increased mortality in 2020 across most nations worldwide, the U.S. had a significantly higher increase compared to other countries. This was also the case for the U.S. in 2021 while mortality declined in most peer nations worldwide. Life expectancy in the U.S. rebounded slightly since the peak of the COVID-19 pandemic but remains far below peer countries.

Premature death rates in the U.S. continue to be higher than in comparable countries. Racial disparities primarily account for the higher rate of premature deaths within the U.S. Specifically, the premature death rates for American Indian and Alaskan Native, Black, Hispanic, Native Hawaiian, and other Pacific Islander populations in the U.S. were 3 times higher than the rates among the White or Asian population. Historically, the U.S. health system consistently results in higher rates of mortality and premature deaths among people of color. Children and teens in the U.S. are less likely to make it to adulthood than in peer countries, with the U.S. having a higher rate of motor vehicle accidents, firearm deaths, and suicide deaths among children and teens.

Maternal mortality rates in the U.S. are much higher than in peer countries. This is a sad irony since in general, wealth and economic prosperity are highly correlated with lower maternal mortality rates. The opposite is true in the U.S. The U.S. has the highest rate of pregnancy-related deaths (22.3 deaths per 100,000 live births) in 2022 when compared to peer countries (3.9 deaths per 100.000 live births). Of note, the maternal mortality rate for Black mothers is significantly higher than the rate for White mothers. Postoperative complications such as pulmonary embolism and deep vein thrombosis are more common in the U.S. than in most peer countries. The U.S. has the highest rates of reported medication and treatment errors than most peer countries. Furthermore, the U.S. has higher rates of consultations missed due to costs than other comparable countries in 2020. (71)

It is easy to see why the U.S. healthcare system is like a sinking ship similar to the Titanic, which everyone thought was virtually unsinkable. And like the Titanic, no one seems to even pay attention to or know how to reverse the downward spiral. Yet, some things can be done. When a patient is in critical condition, a physician first tries to optimize life-saving measures including maintaining good heart function, respirations, good blood flow, and as normal a level of consciousness as possible. Then, as the patient improves, a good physician targets the root of the problem to help the patient fully recover. Likewise, the U.S. healthcare system is in critical condition and in dire need of lifesaving measures to be immediately implemented. Once the patient is stabilized, a good physician strives to identify the cause of the problems so that targeted treatment can be used to reverse an inevitable fatality. In the next chapter, we will get to the root of the problem and discuss possible solutions.

Chapter 9: The Root of The Evil and Perhaps the Way Out

In the case of U.S. health care, lifesaving measures would include efforts to counter physician burnout. Why? Because burnout is causing many good doctors to leave the field and scaring many potentially good doctors from coming into the field. This burnout runs deep and affects all ages, from young medical students, all the way to physicians who are contemplating early retirement. One of the main reasons for burnout is because physicians are no longer allowed to be physicians. In other words, the reason why most doctors become doctors is because they want to take care of patients. Also, most physicians love the autonomy of the profession, which includes making decisions that are in the best interest of the patient based on their knowledge and experience. Autonomy also includes being your own boss, working as much or as little as you want, and pushing yourself to walk the extra mile for others, not because you have to…but because you want to. These are the very reasons why most physicians became physicians, especially those who are older and more experienced. Unfortunately, those days are gone and the sad reality is that these precious assets have been robbed from today's medical doctor. Where does the blame lie?

There are many directions the finger of blame could point to. But one overwhelming path lies in the direction of consolidation. This refers to the ever-increasing efforts by private equity and even by some third-party insurers to pursue mergers and acquisitions of physician-owned clinics and for-profit hospitals. The goal is to dominate the healthcare industry by transforming the previously autonomous physician into an obedient salaried employee. Almost 80% of U.S. physicians are currently employed by hospitals or private companies. (72) This includes third-party insurers like United Health Care which employs 10% of these physicians. Community pharmacies have been replaced by private companies like CVS, Walgreens, and Walmart. Two-thirds of skilled nursing facilities have been taken over by nursing home chains. Health insurance is dominated by five or six large companies. About twelve drug companies produce and dictate the price of the most common prescription medications.

A notable example of the consequences of private equity investment was a large hospital chain known as Steward Healthcare. This chain attempted to expand aggressively outside of Massachusetts by using funding generated from sales-leaseback arrangements with Real Estate Investment Trusts (REITs). The result was a bankruptcy and tremendous harm to the communities the hospitals served. Many private equity firms that own acute care hospitals are engaged in similar practices. A recent study of private equity-owned hospitals showed that 61% of them had significantly reduced capital assets two years after the purchase compared to only 15.5% of controls. Private equity firms that own hospitals prioritize their occupancy rate, not value-based care. Academic medical centers are acquiring more community hospitals as referral sources. Medicare's unfair policy of paying more to hospital outpatient departments than to independent practices has forced many of these practices to either go out of business or to be sold to hospitals owned by private equity.

Pharmaceutical companies have been able to raise prices routinely for patented medications without attempts to negotiate or by lawmakers to regulate. The popular GLP-1 inhibitors prescribed for weight loss and Diabetes may cost the U.S. healthcare system as much as $1 trillion a year. The U.S. spends almost three times as much per person on prescription medications as other developed countries. Justification for such high costs is that pharmaceuticals contend an inability to develop lifesaving medications if their profits are compromised (73) Private equity corporations have one primary goal: to maximize profits. Therefore, private equity in healthcare is a dangerous combination that will only lower the quality of healthcare to the detriment of the patient, the physician, and the U.S. taxpayer. The negative impact of lack of patient access to high-quality health care as well as the rapidly rising cost of health care has trickled down to physician residents in training and even to medical students.

Another direction the finger of blame could point to is the third-party insurers, namely health insurance companies. This entity is responsible for much of the mayhem created in the day-to-day physician's work. Many times, physicians are forced to hire or to contract out for separate staff for billing or dealing with some other aspect of requirements of third-party insurers. For example, these so-called "managed care" third-party health insurers maximize profits by manipulating the system: they use provider networks, prior authorization requirements for prescriptions medications or specialty referrals by health insurance companies, high deductibles and other methods to limit patient access to care and to limit payments to physicians or other providers for services rendered to the patient. These "managed care" tactics consume valuable physician time as well as the time of the physician's staff.

Of course, the same is true with regard to hospitals and large clinics. Yet, the time spent by physicians and their staff satisfying these requirements goes uncompensated by these same insurers. For example, a common health insurance tactic is to offer their clients an annual physical free of charge at any primary care outpatient facility or clinic. The big losers are both the patient and the physician. The reason is that a physician is usually so poorly compensated by the private insurer for this type of examination, that they spend little if any time with the patient in performing it. This means that the quality of a good annual health assessment including a detailed history, review of systems, family history, physical examination, and care recommendations is usually bottled into a 10-15 minute or less interview. The physician usually ends the session by telling the patient that lab work will be ordered. The private health insurer prohibits a physician from using a billing code for a more extensive evaluation after they have seen the patient once. Most patients view this as a benefit in that they can see a doctor for the first visit for free. Yet, the patient is unaware that they are being shortchanged with regard to their health care and that the doctor is being grossly underpaid.

These third-party health insurers are steeped in fraud. Nefarious behavior by third-party health insurers has been documented since as early as 2005 when a confidential audit of 22 Medicare Advantage plans was performed. This audit showed that 31% of the patients were alleged to have diseases by Medicare Advantage plans that could not be confirmed and for which Medicare was paying. Projected losses due to overpayments to Medicare in 2005 alone were $4.2 billion. According to the Center for Medicare Services (CMS), Medicare Advantage overpayments have been linked to the use of a complex "high-risk" formula used to pay for the plans which has virtually no regulations. This formula has been manipulated by Medicare Advantage plans to fraudulently obtain these overpayments via a so-called "honor system". Audits conducted by CMS known as Risk Adjustment Data Validation (RADV) dating back to 2008 estimated overpayment losses to Medicare Advantage plans to be nearly $7 billion. Fraud and abuse by Medicare Advantage plans prompted CMS under Health and Human Services (HHS) to spend $17 million a year simply to conduct RADV audits. These audits turned out to be well worth it because in March 2015 HHS announced that fraud recovery efforts returned $770 for every $1 spent! (74)

Medicare Advantage plans had an improper payment rate estimated at 10% in 2016 costing taxpayers $16.2 billion. Factoring in overpayments by the standard Medicare program to Medicare Advantage plans caused the total amount of abuse to rise to nearly $60 billion in 2016. This is almost twice as much as the National Institute of Health spent on medical research in that same year. (75). More recently, Medicare Advantage plans have enrolled more than 18 million elderly and disabled people. Only about a third of these are eligible for Medicare at a cost to U.S. taxpayers of more than $150 billion a year. (76).

Even more notorious is what was uncovered by the U.S. Senate Permanent Subcommittee Investigation: the three largest Medicare Advantage insurers in the U.S. obstruct seniors' ability to receive post-acute care. It was found that between 2019 and 2022, United Healthcare, CVS, and Humana denied claims for post-acute care at "far higher" rates than for other types of care in 2022. Humana denials in post-acute care were sixteen times higher than the company's overall denial rate. Both United Healthcare and CVS denials were three times higher in the same year. Artificial intelligence was employed to facilitate these denials. The vast majority of the claims were submitted by primary care physicians who cared for these individuals and were seeking compensation for the services provided. Insurance companies base their denial on claims that prior authorization is necessary to prevent unnecessary medical services. But the truth is that these tactics of denial of needed care to seniors are employed by third-party health insurers to maximize their profits. Instead of this practice being outlawed, the sad irony is that it has expanded in recent years. (77)

Another major factor contributing to physician burnout is low pay. This is especially true with regard to primary care physicians. Most people would think this could not possibly be the case with physicians in general. But just think about it. What other profession is forced to accept payment by their clients at a hugely discounted rate from government programs? What other profession is obligated to accept payment by their clients from private health insurers whose fee schedules mimic the government programs? What other profession has experienced a steady decline in the rate of pay for virtually 23 consecutive years representing a 29% total reduction in pay? What other profession faces in addition to the past cuts in payment, a looming 2.8% cut in the Medicare Physician Fee Schedule (MPFS) already mandated to begin January 1, 2025, representing a total almost 33% pay cut? What other profession is forced to depend on huge corporate entities like third party health insurers for their income within a strange employer-employee relationship?

In this relationship, the mythical "employer" is the third-party health insurer who has the option to either deny payment or to give partial payment without justifiable cause to the "employee". The mythical "employee" is the physician and staff. On the other hand, the "employer" may choose to heavily discount what is paid to the "employee" from their usual rates for the services provided and to deny the physician's account of the time involved in caring for their mutual client. Furthermore, what other profession is obligated to devote the time of their staff as well as themselves to fulfill the requirements of these corporate entities? Yet, this is all expected by the "employer" to be done by the "employee" free of charge with no compensation whatsoever for the time or resources involved nor for coverage of any overhead expenses. What other profession is abandoned to the mercy or lack thereof of nefarious private health insurers' practices without government regulation or oversight? The obvious answer is physicians. In stark contrast, lawyers, accountants, engineers, and architects among other professions, can charge and exact an hourly rate for their services according to the time they claim to have spent.

The payment cuts to the Medicare Physician Fee Schedule have recently come to the attention of lawmakers in Congress who are alarmed at the ripple effects this is having on the healthcare sector, in particular physicians. A recently submitted bipartisan letter signed by 233 House members stated the following: "Increased instability in the health care sector due to looming cost hikes impacts the ability of physicians and clinicians to provide the highest quality of care and threatens patient access to affordable healthcare". The letter went on to state: "instead of these harmful cuts, which absent federal legislation, will take effect on January 1, 2025, Congress must pass a bill providing physicians and other clinicians with a payment update that takes into account the cost of actually delivering care to patients". The negative impact of these continual Medicare payment cuts on the healthcare sector has been enormous: medical groups and integrated systems of care have been forced to impose hiring freezes, delay system improvements, and delay implementation of care model changes including translations to value-based care systems and in some cases, eliminating services. These members of Congress also expressed concerns for needed reform in the mandated Medicare Physician Fee Schedule (MPFS) budget neutrality requirements which fails to take into account cost increases due to inflation, cost of living, and rising practice expense costs. Furthermore, the Center for Medicare Services was mandated to limit changes to the MPFS conversion factor to no more than 2.5% in a given year. (78). The problem is amplified in that third-party health insurers copy the Medicare Physician Fee Schedule as a basis of their payments to physicians. Yet, third-party health insurers also routinely deny payments to physicians due to unjustifiable claims of "no medical necessity" or they pay at rates lower than the Medicare Physician Fee Schedule. Yet, the third-party health insurers are given free rein to raise their premiums annually to their clients and as a result, they reap huge profits.

Primary care physicians are especially targeted for lower pay. These are lumped into one category for simplification of payment purposes by both Medicare/Medicaid and third-party insurers. As previously mentioned, primary care includes Physician Assistants, Nurse Practitioners in primary care, General practitioners who have only one year of residency training beyond medical school, Family practitioners with a more general three-year residency training, Pediatricians with a three-year residency training in caring for the medical problems of children, adolescents and newborns and Internal Medicine physicians who have a three-year residency training in caring for the medical problems of adults. Even though the latter two physician categories are considered specialties, both Medicare/Medicaid and private insurers group them into the category of primary care providers as opposed to specialist providers, who are placed in a separate, more privileged category. However primary care providers are given much lower payments for their services. Why? Because, since its inception, Medicare has traditionally placed greater value on surgery and medical procedures than on methodical history taking, physical examination, review of labs, and imaging reports to make an accurate diagnosis and to prescribe correct treatments. The latter are the very activities that Internal Medicine physicians and Pediatricians spend the bulk of their time on in patient care.

The reason for this biased viewpoint is largely due to the influence of the American Medical Association (AMA), which is controlled primarily by surgeons. This group advises Medicare annually regarding reimbursement to providers. Also, little value is placed on the diagnostic methods employed by the primary care physician, especially Internal Medicine physicians. These methods include obtaining detailed family and social histories to isolate certain risk factors so that preventative measures can be employed to mitigate and prevent disease and suffering in the future. On the other hand, "specialists" include surgeons, surgical subspecialists, and medical subspecialist providers who perform procedures. Private health insurers mimic the fee schedule of Medicare annually and at times, may pay less than the Medicare fee schedule.

This is especially true in the case of primary care providers. For example, I was recently compensated by a third health party insurer for only $8 for multiple prescription refills. This rate of pay is well below minimum wage. Primary care physicians are forced to expect low pay while inflation in 2023 was at an all-time high, the cost of living continues to rise, practice expenses are spiraling out of control and patients are conditioned to pay for their doctor visits only with their insurance without further out-of-pocket expense. Also, Medicare, Medicaid, and third-party private insurers will only pay for limited-time follow-up visits, usually no more than three to four per year, traditionally for less than fifteen minutes. This is why physicians must see a huge volume of patients to maintain a sustainable income. Otherwise, they will be forced into a fiscal crisis which will inevitably end in the closure or sale of their practice. The bottom line is that Medicare has been paying specialists too much and primary care providers too little for years. Third-party health insurers have followed the same practice which has caused a huge income gap between primary care providers and specialists. (79)

These causes of burnout were greatly amplified during and after the COVID-19 pandemic. Major weaknesses of the U.S. health care system were exposed during this period which almost virtually collapsed when it was most needed. Also, the pandemic brought about an even greater impetus for young physicians to become sub-specialists or surgeons to survive. As a result, talented physicians previously in primary care, have departed in droves. No wonder medical students who face huge medical school debt see no other viable path forward than to pursue a subspecialty career. All the while, the primary care physician workforce continues to shrink. It seems that corporate entities and perhaps some lawmakers have the unrealistic hope that physicians will eventually be replaced by non-physician practitioners or possibly, all will be replaced by artificial intelligence. Thus, we now have a predominant specialist-oriented health care system where if one has common medical problems, they are mandated to see a specialist. For example, if you have an earache, you have to see an ENT specialist….if you have a cough, you have to see a pulmonologist……if you have a headache, you have to see a neurologist. This type of care is dramatically raising the cost of health care and at the same time, is exasperating and confusing the patient who is passed around like a football from one physician to another.

This move to replace physicians with non-physicians was highlighted recently in the state of Vermont. A recent state-commissioned report recommended major reductions in service at four small Vermont hospitals.

THE DECIMATION OF U.S. HEALTHCARE

The recommendations included converting inpatient beds to mental health care, changing emergency department staffing to a non-physician model, and moving obstetric services outside the hospital. The report said that without major restructuring, 13 of Vermont's 14 hospitals will be operating at a loss by 2028. The report added that 9 of Vermont's hospitals were already operating in the red financially in 2023. The report concluded that if nothing is done in the next 3-5 years, hospitals, citizens, or both would face bankruptcy. A leader of the state chapter of the American College of Emergency Physicians issued public letters earlier in autumn 2024 opposing the report's recommendation to convert emergency departments to non-physician models, citing safety concerns. Specifically, the letter stated: "As written, this recommendation threatens the quality of health care delivery in Vermont and the safety and well-being of Vermonters."(80) This trend to save money by compromising health care is happening all over the country. Therefore, one reality is very clear: the quality of U.S. health care has dramatically declined especially over the last three decades and is continuing on a rapid downward spiral.

So, is there any hope for this sinking ship known as U.S. health care? Will the ship completely sink? In other words, will the decimation of U.S. health care continue until the system completely collapses? Probably, unless drastic measures are taken. Going back to the illustration of a critical patient, a good physician will first try to maintain life-sustaining measures, such as optimizing the patient's vital signs. Once achieved, a good physician will try to analyze and find the cause of the problem to administer targeted specific treatment to relieve suffering and ultimately, to cure the patient from their ailment. When this happens, everyone benefits.

THE DECIMATION OF U.S. HEALTHCARE

Not only will the patient survive, but also the physician will feel a sense of true accomplishment and value.

Just as a good doctor must be able to recognize what the problem is that the patient is suffering to be able to successfully treat and cure them, one must recognize the problem with the U.S. healthcare system to improve it and to have the possibility of saving it from total collapse. One has to first recognize that medicine is a unique profession in which physicians must devote a lifelong dedication to their work. All new physicians are required to swear to the Hippocratic oath to uphold ethical standards. These standards include treating patients to the best of one's ability and judgment, avoiding harm to patients or causing injustice, and avoiding corruption or impropriety to patients. (81).

In the past, the vast majority of physicians have had no problem with keeping this oath throughout a lifetime of practice. Yet, currently, we have a healthcare system of physicians who are "unevenly yoked" with corporate greed. U.S. health care has developed into a strange form of socialized medicine that has become subjected to and dominated by a capitalist society. In other words, the altruistic autonomous practice of Medicine has become dominated by corporate entities that only have the goal of making more profit. These corporate entities have no concerns regarding the quality of health care rendered, nor concerns about patient outcomes, survival, or patient or physician costs. The principal concern is the most effective way to maximize profits. As long as corporate entities are allowed to profit from healthcare, the result will be an even lower quality of healthcare delivered, worse healthcare outcomes, shorter average life expectancy for the recipients, and increased costs passed on to the patient along with an ever-dwindling number of physicians administering care.

Since primary care is the backbone of any health care system which has already been broken in the U.S., a vigorous effort can and should be made to mend it. How? Currently, the U.S. only devotes 5% of its healthcare budget and less than 5% of Medicare spending to primary care. This is even though primary care accounts for more than 35% of healthcare visits. This has been the case since 2012. (82),(83). This figure should be dramatically increased at least to correspond with the pivotal role primary care plays as the very foundation of the health care system. Increasing primary care physicians' compensation substantially would attract more talented physicians to the field instead of driving them away, as has been the case for many years. Also, primary care physicians should be compensated in the same manner as other professions, like accountants and attorneys: in accord with their level of expertise, education, and experience.

Internal Medicine physicians and Pediatricians are specialists in the field of chronic medical care for adults and children respectively, and they deserve to be paid for their level of expertise. Attorneys and accountants working in private practice or for firms can exact an hourly wage for their services. Many even charge at 6-minute intervals and submit invoices to their clients expecting commensurate payment for all the time claimed. It is only fair that physicians in private practice in primary care be paid for the time spent caring for each patient. However, the current system in place with Medicare and third-party health insurers does not recognize this right to be compensated for the time spent. Both, reserve the right to deny payment altogether or to grossly underpay what is charged by the physician. The former may have some limited justification in that it is a federal government program funded by taxpayers. However, the latter is a for-profit entity determined to pay the physician as little as possible to maximize their profits. Also, the practice of categorizing physicians as a primary care provider or specialist should be discarded. This practice, adopted by Medicare to simplify payment, has grossly cheated physicians, especially Internal Medicine physicians and Pediatricians. These, who are considered specialists by their residency training, are paid by Medicare and third-party health insurers at the same rate as nonphysician practitioners.

As mentioned, once a good physician stabilizes a patient, he seeks to find the cause of the problem to administer the appropriate curative treatment. In looking back on the history of the downward spiral of U.S. health care, one obvious cause is greed. Greed by corporate entities, including third-party insurers and other corporate giants, which seek to make huge profits from the healthcare industry is the root of the problem. Like a glutton who takes in overwhelmingly more calories than are burned in exercise, the expected result will be to become fatter and fatter. Likewise, this is how third-party health insurers and private equity have become….fatter and fatter. The goal of both entities is to take in as much money as possible and to pay out as little as possible to reap huge profits. This was originally the case with third-party health insurers.

These corporate entities have gone either unregulated or poorly regulated in this country which has allowed them to freely operate as legalized scams. Unfortunately, the wary victims of these legalized scams include both patients and physicians. The patient is being robbed of possibly life-saving and potentially suffering sparing preventative care. Simultaneously, the patient has been stuck with the bills of higher health care costs. On the other hand, physicians are robbed of compensation due to their skills, education, experience, and expertise which took a lifetime to develop. Not to mention, they are also deprived of the autonomy and satisfaction of caring for others which are privileges unique to their profession.

Why are physicians in the U.S. forced to work as indentured servants? Why are they obligated to be either grossly underpaid or at times, not paid at all? Yet, all this takes place in a capitalist society. This situation is amplified in the case of primary care physicians. Most primary care private practices are virtually unsustainable given rising overhead practice costs and the cost of living to deal with monthly. Also, why does the federal government allow third-party health insurers to privatize taxpayer-funded government programs like Medicare and Medicaid? It is understandable why private health insurers would seize the opportunity to profit from Medicaid. They were readily informed that starting in 2014, billions of dollars in Medicaid revenues would be available nationwide for managed-care plans as a result of the ACA's Medicaid expansion. (84)

Both Medicare and Medicaid were meant to benefit elderly, disabled, and low-income Americans and now provide coverage for more than 40% of the U.S. population. Yet, as of 2022, 48% of Medicare beneficiaries were enrolled in Medicare Advantage plans compared to only 25% just 10 years prior. Two private health insurers, United Health Care and Humana alone, account for almost half of all Medicare Advantage enrollment. As of 2020, 72% of Medicaid beneficiaries were enrolled in managed care plans dominated by only five insurance companies: United Health Care, Centene, Anthem (renamed "Elevance Health" in 2022, Molina, and Aetna/CVS accounting for half of all enrollment. These public programs are now a principal source of revenue for health insurance companies. A recent analysis by KFF (Kaiser Family Foundation) found that gross margins per enrollee defined as the amount by which total premium income exceeds total claims costs per person over a specified period (per year), were higher in 2021 for both Medicare Advantage and Medicaid managed care than for employer-sponsored insurance. The gross margin per enrollee for Medicare Advantage was $1730 and Medicaid managed care was $768, while it was $689 for employer-sponsored insurance. Figures like this prompted Humana to announce that it was leaving the employer market and would instead give undivided attention to the Medicare and Medicaid sectors. (85). The fact is that Medicare Advantage plans have both higher average costs and higher premiums which are largely paid for by the federal government. The justification is due to Medicare covering the health care of an older, sicker population. For this reason, gross margins per enrollee in Medicare Advantage plans tend to be higher which means third-party health insurers' profit and administrative costs are also higher.

This makes sense for private health insurance companies. The Medicare Payment Advisory Committee estimates that the government overpays Medicare Advantage plans 6% more than would have been paid for beneficiaries in traditional Medicare. The net result was that $27 billion in excess spending went to private health insurers in 2023. This gross overpayment is largely the result of the private insurer's mastery of using the risk adjustment score to inflate the number of medical diagnoses of each enrollee to receive higher reimbursement. Private health insurers also utilized prior authorization to lower their costs substantially. This tactic is primarily used for specialty care, imaging, and pharmaceuticals to avoid payment for care seen by them as inappropriate or medically unnecessary. Yet, for patients and physicians, prior authorization adds tremendous administrative burden and impediments to care. (86).

Private health insurers have been given free rein to take advantage of federal government programs while amassing huge profits. But, why is it that the very providers of health care are often overlooked, underpaid, or not paid at all, while third-party health insurers are paid excessively? Why are physicians forced to accept commercial insurance as a payment from patients along with the obligatory huge discounts from their charges that this acceptance entails? The decision of whether or not to accept payment at a discounted rate from government tax payer funded programs such as Medicare and Medicaid are one that every physician will have to determine. Yet, why are physicians forced to accept discounted rates from private insurance companies who are reaping huge profits at the physician's expense? On the other hand, third-party health insurers are not willing to discount their annual premium charges to their clients. Is this not a double standard? Not to mention the fact that the physician is unaware at the time of the visit whether the payment will be made by the insurance company, the patient, or by neither. The latter is the case when the insurance company says "the bill is the patient's responsibility" due to the deductible not being met, but the patient still refuses to pay. Or the patient may only come for a physician visit expecting to get a free annual exam promised by the insurance company and decline any further appointments. On the other hand, the insurance company may refuse to pay, citing unjustifiably that there was "no medical necessity" for the visit.

Furthermore, a ridiculously complex formula concocted by Medicare has been employed to place a dollar value on a physician's care. This bizarre and esoteric formula favors surgeons and medical subspecialists but short-changes primary care physicians. This is especially true regarding Internal Medicine physicians, who make decisions routinely to manage and prevent chronic disease. Third-party health insurers have followed suit by adopting the same fee-for-service structure instituted by Medicare to enrich themselves to the detriment of the patient and the physician. Also, third-party health insurers have learned how to manipulate the patient risk score used to receive monthly capitated payments from Medicare. They have masterminded deceptive tactics to increase the patient's diagnosis codes. This is done because they know that the sicker the patient is listed as being, the greater the monthly capitated payment received from Medicare will be. This is pertinent in that Medicare is the costliest public health insurance program in the world and it makes up a significant portion of U.S. government spending. One study showed that conservative estimates of overpayments to Medicare Advantage plans amounted to $10.2 billion a year. (87)

Unfortunately, this fraud also means a much higher bill for the American taxpayer and in most cases, even for the patient. Nevertheless, the patient does not receive better care, and in most cases, the health outcome and survival are worse than with traditional Medicare.

Third-party insurers are also profiting significantly from the Affordable Care Act. Annual premiums are adjusted lower for older sicker people, but much higher for younger healthier people. Especially is this true in the case of young men. (88). These higher premiums are largely paid for by taxpayer subsidies known as "premium tax credits". A record 92% of marketplace enrollees or 19.7 million people qualified for premium tax credits in 2024. These premium tax credits allowed people with incomes between 100-150% of the poverty level to pay $0 in annual premiums for "benchmark" silver plans. Even those with incomes above 400% of the poverty level were extended eligibility for premium tax credits if the benchmark premiums exceeded 8.5% of their household income. As a result, the average enrollee in ACA saved $700 in 2024 due to premium tax credits. (89) Despite the taxpayer-funded subsidies, premiums are raised annually by third-party insurers, with no questions asked. Also, third-party insurers have infiltrated states that offer Medicaid expansion to fleece that market, further ripping off the federal government and taxpayers.

What can and should be done about this? Medicare and Medicaid should eliminate their marriage with third-party health insurers. Private health insurance companies should be completely separate from federal government programs designed to promote public health. The results of this uneven alliance have been disastrous for both the patient and the physician. Third-party health insurers, who provide no direct care for the patient, should no longer receive capitated monthly payments from Medicare. Instead, primary care physicians, especially Internal Medicine physicians, and Pediatricians, who provide direct care to the patient, should receive monthly capitated payments depending on the number and the state of health of the patients seen.

An alternative method of payment would be for Medicare to pay primary care physicians at an hourly rate stipulated by each clinician according to their level of education, experience, and the time involved in caring for each patient. Medical subspecialists and surgeons should be paid in the same manner, according to the procedure or surgery performed, commensurate with the level of their education and experience. However, they should not be paid disproportionately more than primary care physicians. On the other hand, third-party insurers should provide health coverage to the patient based on revenues generated by annual premiums alone, as is the case with other private insurance company sectors. Similar to other insurance carriers, private third-party health insurers should use their capital, not the federal government's, to insure patients. Also, private health insurance should only be used for coverage of hospitalization, emergent or urgent care, procedures, surgeries, or medications. It should not be used by the patient to pay for medical office visits. This method of payment has been a millstone around the neck and a pitfall for physicians over the years. All too often, the physician, especially the primary care physician, is left to be the one taking the financial loss. For example, a patient presents his insurance for payment for a visit with a physician. After submission of the claim, the insurance company declares that the entire amount which has been significantly discounted from the physician's original charge, is the patient's responsibility. But, the patient refuses to pay the balance even though they were satisfied with the care rendered. Third-party insurers are quick to deny payments to physicians using billing codes that give credit for the physician spending longer periods devoted to patient care. Also, denials or gross underpayments are routinely made for such things as electrocardiograms performed for patients complaining of chest pain or for prescription refill requests. This is done without explanation or justification. Also, third-party insurers deny payment to physicians citing "no medical necessity" without contemporary physician review or with legal regulation. While practice costs have steadily risen, inflation rates recently at an all-time high, along with the cost of living increasing daily, physicians have been saddled with a nearly 32% reduction in payment by Medicare and third-party health insurers over the last 23 years. It may be in part, understandable to accept reduced payments from federal programs. Yet, to do so is inexplicable in the case of capitalist-minded private health insurers, who only seek their company's advantage. No longer should a physician's income or patient care depend upon profiteering third-party health insurers.

Third-party insurers should not be allowed to profit from Medicaid or the Affordable Care Act. Furthermore, third-party health insurers should be restricted from imposing "managed care" requirements upon patients and physicians. This so-called "managed care" really implies "mismanaged care" and possibly "no care" at all, implemented by non-physician personnel. Eliminating the third-party insurer from the equation would mean the end of burdensome administrative requirements imposed by these entities. Such requirements not only unnecessarily drive up the cost of health care, but also take valuable time away from patient care. Prior Authorization is another tactic of third-party insurers that robs valuable time from the physician and his staff. This time goes uncompensated by third-party insurers. Also, prior authorization can deprive patients of needed surgery, procedures, or medications.

The record of third-party health insurers are evident. Comparisons of traditional Medicare with Medicare Advantage plans clearly show that not only is the American taxpayer being fleeced to the tune of billions of dollars, but the recipients of this care have worse outcomes, including higher rates of mortality and morbidity.

Private equity should also be no part of health care in the U.S. Their greed rivals the gluttonous attitude of the third-party insurers. This greed has made U.S. health care more dangerous to the public than ever. Medicine is a science and an art, not a commodity. The greedy private equity companies see health care as a commodity that if produced in large quantities, will reap even greater profit. However, the human body is not a commodity. Instead, it is enormously complex, and at the same time, very fragile. If you want to build a house, you will need an architect. On the other hand, if you want to tear a house down, you may only need a carpenter or perhaps, a demolition team. Internal Medicine doctors are like architects, who approach the human body with tremendous respect for its complexity. Yet, at the same time, they are keenly aware of the human body's fragility. This is especially the case as a person ages. This is why, at times, hours are spent unraveling a mysterious disease, or perhaps a condition, that masquerades with a unique manifestation. However private equity has no regard for the life-changing aspects of diagnostic acumen involved in masterful patient care. The instruction for the physician instead, is to spend as little time as possible with each patient and to see as many people as possible within a finite period. If the physician is not able or willing to comply with this direction, the physician is subject to be replaced or terminated. Private equity will not hesitate to replace the physicians with cheaper nonphysician practitioners. And if deemed by them as feasible in the future, perhaps all health care practitioners may be replaced with artificial intelligence.

Replacement of physicians has already happened in many emergency rooms across the U.S. and in the Veteran's Administration Center. The situation in many emergency rooms throughout the U.S. has almost become similar to the uncertainty associated with being in a car without a driver. You or your loved one may arrive at a hospital emergency room or an Urgent Care facility automatically assuming that the care will be provided by a physician qualified to handle emergencies. Yet, increasingly in the U.S., people will be evaluated and treated by a nonphysician practitioner rather than a physician when going to an emergency room or an urgent care facility. Already, most urgent care facilities throughout the U.S. are only staffed by nonphysician practitioners.

Experts say nurse practitioners are taking the place of doctors in many urgent care clinics and emergency rooms. Nurse practitioner and physician assistant training programs were originally developed to train individuals to function under the supervision of physicians, thus extending the ability of the physician to provide service to a greater number of patients. However, in many areas, these nonphysician practitioners are allowed full practice authority without the supervision of a physician. Doctors say that there is little incentive among profit-seeking companies, especially urgent care facilities, to keep paying doctors when they can hire nurse practitioners and substantially cut costs. Yet, a 2013 Mayo Clinic study compared the quality of referrals of patients with complex medical problems from nurse practitioners, physician assistants, and physicians. The results of the study showed the quality of referrals to an academic medical center was higher for physicians than for nurse practitioners and physician assistants with regard to the clarity of the referral question, the understanding of the pathophysiology, adequacy of pre-referral evaluation, and documentation. Furthermore, the AMA maintains the position that while nurse practitioners and other mid-level medical workers are an important part of the medical team, they are not a substitute for physicians in diagnosing complex medical problems.

The concern among physicians for unsupervised nonphysician practice has inspired the development of Physicians for Patient Protection (PPP). This is a group of physicians, residents, and medical students whose mission is to ensure physician-led care for patients and to advocate for truth and transparency regarding healthcare practitioners. Groups like this reflect a growing number of physicians who feel that patients are being harmed by nonphysicians working without physician supervision and that this is contributing to the astronomical costs of health care in the U.S.(90). This means that any of us could become unfortunate victims if we suddenly needed emergent or urgent care or happened to be a veteran.

Yet, alternative methods of caring for patients by physicians are popping up all over the country. For, example, many primary care physicians, especially Internal Medicine physicians, have switched to concierge practices. Survey results showed that it would take more than 24 hours a day for doctors to follow nationally recommended guidelines for preventative care, chronic disease care management, and acute care visits. This time frame is due to the average number of patients seen in a usual primary care practice. Yet, the average doctor visit currently only lasts 18 minutes according to a National Institute of Health finding. On the other hand, a physician within a concierge practice takes care of a much smaller panel of patients daily and weekly.

These patients generally have much greater access to their physician, which in some cases can extend to 24/7 coverage. Their care includes an in-depth physical exam and preventative screening tests. The patient agrees to an annual membership contract in which the physician is paid either annually or monthly. Physicians also continue to accept and bill the patient's insurance plan or government program for covered services. Concierge practices tend to be more popular and accepted in high-income populations.

Another model of practice that is rapidly emerging is known as Direct Patient Care (DPC). This model has especially been rising in popularity among Family Practice physicians. Physicians operating within this type of practice do not accept third-party insurance. Thus, insurance-related staffing expenses are eliminated along with burdensome administrative insurance requirements.

This means that the physician no longer needs staff to manage administrative requirements of third-party insurers such as prior authorization or billing through clearing houses. The benefits include significantly fewer overhead costs as well as lower costs to the patient for diagnostic tests, prescription medications, and even referrals to medical subspecialists or surgeons. The reason is that the physician can negotiate lower rates for all these services. The physician is paid a monthly or annual fee that is generally more affordable than in concierge practices. Similar to concierge practices, physicians in DPC practice have a significantly decreased patient panel and can therefore focus more on giving quality care. They are free of the burden of seeing as many patients as possible hastily.

This type of practice fosters the development of a stronger relationship between the physician with patients, greatly simplifies billing, and creates a more pleasant environment, eliminating the likelihood of physician burnout. The patients benefit in that they feel that they receive more individualized and personal care. They also have extended time with the physician and most patients feel they have better access to the physician either in person or by phone. However, it is prudent for the patient to have additional insurance coverage with these models of practice. Usually, it is best to acquire a high-deductible wrap-around insurance policy, with either model of practice.

Additional insurance would provide coverage in the event of emergencies, especially requiring hospitalization. These ancillary policies also are beneficial to have in the event of the need to see subspecialist physicians, or surgeons or to cover the cost of prescription medications. Furthermore, many of the health care costs not covered by a Direct Primary Care or Concierge medicine practice are reimbursable through an employer with a Health Reimbursement Arrangement (HRA). These plans allow employers to reimburse their employees tax-free for qualifying medical expenditures. (91) There are also hybrid models of patient care that have developed with combinations of the above. Some physicians who are in private practices in a clinic setting charge hourly rates and others only accept cash or credit cards without accepting insurance. The trend is moving far away from third-party health insurers and corporate greed to deliver quality care to patients.

. When people are dissatisfied with their work situation, usually concerning compensation, working conditions, or both, they form coalitions to protest. Unions are formed and workers threaten to leave their jobs in the form of strikes unless their demands are met. Even healthcare workers, usually nurses, have resorted to these tactics. But the fact is that most doctors are neither sufficiently organized nor united to form unions. Instead, doctors have chosen to deal with professional grievances as individuals or through membership organizations like the American College of Physicians or the American College of Emergency Physicians. When faced with burnout, many physicians, residents in training and even some medical students have chosen to change their career goals to another profession. Others have chosen to pursue early retirement or simply retire. If this trend continues at the current pace, physicians will eventually be completely replaced by non-physician practitioners and the quality of health care will dramatically decline.

It is obvious that drastic measures must be taken now to reverse the course of U.S. healthcare. While the U.S. has the most expensive health care of any country in the world, medical debt is the most common reason for bankruptcy. In fact, 66.5% of the bankruptcies in the U.S. are caused directly by medical expenses. This is the case even though most of the people are insured. (92) Billions of dollars per year of taxpayer funds could be saved by eliminating third-party health insurers from profiting from both Medicare and Medicaid. Health care is being provided by physicians, not by health insurance companies.

Therefore, the physician should be paid for both their services and their time. The Medicare Fee-for-Service arrangement should be abolished. Instead, a value-based payment model should be instituted that would account not only for the physician's time but also for the level of experience and training rendered. A value-based model is more likely to promote measures that would improve care or make it safer. On the other hand, with a fee-for-service model, these incentives are much less likely to exist. (93) Capitated monthly payments from Medicare should be paid to physicians, not to third-party health insurers.

Furthermore, third-party health insurers are fleecing the U.S. government for billions of dollars as a result of overinflated annual premium costs for Medicaid and the Affordable Care Act paid for primarily by taxpayer subsidies. Patients, in turn, either receive poor quality health care or no care at all. Private equity policies are also rapidly driving away quality physicians and replacing them with nonphysician practitioners. Corporate greed has reduced physicians to employees for whom much is demanded and relatively little is paid. Emphasis is placed on the quantity of patients seen as opposed to the quality of care rendered. As a result, the patient receives steadily declining, poorer quality health care, and the physician is driven to a burnout stage. Also, private equity is costing U.S. healthcare billions of dollars per year more than if corporations were not involved. Big business should have no place in healthcare and should be removed from the equation for the benefit of all, but especially, for the benefit of the patient.

Currently, almost 80% of physicians in the U.S. are salaried employees with half of all physician practices owned by a hospital or corporate entity. United Health Group is the country's largest physician employer with 70,000 salaried or affiliated physicians. Retailers such as Amazon, CVS, and Walgreens have spent billions of dollars expanding their primary care in nearly every state. Furthermore, private equity investors have now encompassed more than 30% of certain local markets. Not only are corporate entities dominating health care but there is also a growing concern that corporations are gradually exerting control over clinical operations. This includes management and staffing decisions, billing and coding practices, as well as negotiations with insurers. Control of all of these facets of care by corporate entities is likely to pressure physicians to change care delivery. Therefore, there are three main risks that corporate entities' domination of health care will pose; 1) increased healthcare prices and spending due to market consolidation and exploitation of payment loopholes. 2) patient care concerns associated with changes in practice patterns and pressures to reduce staffing. 3) moral injury and burnout among physicians.

How can states prevent the corporatization of medicine? One way is to strengthen the Corporate Practice of Medicine (CPOM) laws. There are three basic ways to do this. First, states could close existing loopholes that permit corporate ownership. Second, states could regulate the MSO Management Services Organization model. Under this model, corporate entities operate a completely owned management services organization (MSO) that contracts with a medical practice's P.C. The MSO is nominally owned by licensed physicians but is solely managed and operated by the MSO, not by the physicians.

A more extreme version of this MSO model is called the "friendly PC" model. Within this model, a medically licensed executive is appointed as owner, director, and officer of the MSO's target practices. This arrangement allows lay corporations to assume de facto ownership and control of physician practices. The third way states could further prohibit the corporate practice of medicine is by barring physician contracts from including restrictive provisions, such as stock-restriction agreements, noncompete clauses, and broader protection for whistleblowers from retaliation when they cite patient safety or ethical concerns. (94). Unfortunately, these reforms are unlikely to take place within the current atmosphere which favors little to no government regulation.

The sad reality is that while the U.S. has the best doctors in the world, the healthcare system ranks at the bottom of the list of developed countries. Foremost among the reasons is that the quality of coverage is worse in the U.S. than in any other country in the world. Specifically, among Americans with insurance, nearly a quarter are underinsured, facing high deductibles and co-payments that reduce the effectiveness of their insurance in assuring access to needed care. (95) This is particularly problematic in accessing preventative and comprehensive primary care which is the backbone of any good health care system. This is the reason why countries like Taiwan, Singapore, Japan, South Korea, Australia, and Canada are consistently at the top of the list of healthcare systems in the world: they all have a type of universal coverage with third-party health insurers playing a minor, if any role. For example, Taiwan has an efficient single-payer system that provides universal coverage and emphasizes prevention. South Korea is ranked highly due to its advanced technology in health care and a strong national health insurance program. (96) Japan also provides universal coverage that is funded primarily by taxes and individual contributions. All are required to enroll in either an employment-based or a residence-based health insurance plan. Benefits included hospital care, primary care, specialty care, and mental health care along with coverage for prescription drugs. In addition to premiums, citizens pay 30% co-insurance for most services and some co-payments.

Young children and low-income older adults have lower co-insurance rates and there is an annual out-of-pocket maximum for health care and long-term services based on age and income. There are also monthly out-of-pocket maximums. The national government sets the fee schedule and gives subsidies to local governments, including municipalities and prefectures as well as to insurers and providers. The government also establishes and enforces detailed regulations for insurers and providers. Most residents have private health insurance, but it is used primarily as a supplement to life insurance providing additional income in case of illness. (97). This is in stark contrast to the U.S. healthcare system which promotes third-party privatized involvement and zero support for primary care or physicians in private practice.

In conclusion, the U.S. healthcare system is like a sinking ship. The only way to save a sinking ship is to unload much of the cargo. The successful health care systems provide for the people by having some sort of universal coverage free of third-party health insurers' domination. Therefore, third-party health insurers should be banned from federal government programs like Medicare and Medicaid as well as the Affordable Care Act.

Another option is that they would assume a lesser role, such as complementary to life insurance in the event of a major illness, as is the case with Japan's health care system. Physicians should not be obligated to accept huge discounted rates from private health insurers, especially since they are in turn making huge profits. Instead, the rates should be negotiated more equitably, taking into account the time spent with each patient, provided there is mutual agreement between the two parties. Private equity corporations should not be allowed to enter into and dominate health care in the U.S. Instead, corporate entities should be prohibited from owning hospitals and medical practices.

All the data shows that corporate equity involvement in health care leads to higher costs, increased physician burnout, worse health care outcomes, and overall, significantly lower quality of health care. Pharmaceutical companies must have strict price controls imposed by legislators. Tax payers, by means of the federal government, should neither be obligated to subsidize or enrich pharmaceutical companies nor third-party health insurers. Furthermore, it should always be remembered that without a solid foundation, a building will in time, collapse. Likewise, without a solid primary care foundation which is the very backbone of medicine and any good health care system, the health care system will also in time collapse.

Also, there has to be a concerted effort to recruit and support primary care physicians, chief among them, Internal Medicine physicians for adolescents and adults and Pediatricians for infants and children. No longer should private corporations be allowed to view health care as an industry to make a profit and not as a service that is purposed to help people. On the other hand, doctors became doctors because they wanted to give their patients the best quality health care they could. Patients expect and deserve quality health care from their doctors. We all look forward to the time the Bible speaks of in Isaiah 33:24 when "no resident will say: "I am sick". However, until that time comes, and if many of the factors discussed in this book are allowed to persist, it will continue to contribute to the decimation of U.S. healthcare. Yet, just maybe, this outcry will no longer fall on deaf ears. Perhaps, the public will be spared from suffering the collapse of healthcare… from one becoming old and sick, or maybe, young and disabled, with no one to care for them……..How sad that would be. Moreover, perhaps someone, lawmakers or physicians, will somehow find a way to save this health care "ship" from sinking. But this will only happen if someone in authority listens and institutes monumental changes….before it is too late.

References

1. CMS.gov Newsroom, National Health Expenditures 2022 Highlights

2. National Archives, Milestone Documents, Medicare and Medicaid Act (1965)

3. Robin, Rony Caryn. 15-minute Doctor Visits Take a Toll on Patient-Physician Relationships. PBS News

4. Frieben, Joyce. Medicare Finalizes 3.4% Payment Cut For Physician Fees in 2024. Medphage Today.

5. Patel Y.M. and Guterman S. The Evolution of Private Plans in Medicare. Improving Health Care Quality. The Commonwealth Fund. 2017, December 8.

6. Morrisey, M.A. Health Insurance, Second Edition. Chapter 1, page 10.

7. Minemyer, Paige. United Health was 2021's Most Profitable Payer, Here's a Look at What It's Competitors Earned. 2022, February 11.

8. Pifer, Rebecca, United Health Flush off 2022 Momentum, Eyes Membership Value Based Growth. Health Care Dive. Zelis. 2023, January 13.

9. Turner, Ani, Miller, George, Lowry, Elise. High U.S. Health Care Spending: Where is it All Going? Controlling Health Care Costs. The Commonwealth Fund. 2023, October 4.

10. Guinan, Stephanie. Insurance Claim Denials: Worst Companies and How to Appeal. Value Penguin. 2024, May 15.

11. Rucker, Patrick, Miller, Maya, Armstrong, David. How Cigna Saves Millions by Having It's Doctors Reject Claims Without Reading Them. Health Care Propublica

12. Buckner, J.D, Susan. Legally Reviewed by Richmond, Esq. Susan Mills. Health Care and Bad Faith Insurance Claims. Find Law. 2024, May 20.

13. Howley, Elaine. The U.S. Physician Shortage Is Only Going To Get Worse. Here Are Potential Solutions. Time. 2022, July 25.

14. Caplan, Zoe. U.S. Older Population Grew From 2010 to 2020 at Fastest Rate Since 1880 to 1890, 2020 Census: 1 in 6 People in the United States Were 65 and Older. United States Census. 2023, May 25.

15. Get the Facts on Older Americans, Aging in America. National Council on Aging.

16. New AAMC Report Shows Continuing Projected Physician Shortage. Press Release. AAMC

17. Benavidez, G.A., PhD, Zahnd, W.E., PhD, Hung, P., PhD, Eberth, J.M., PhD. Chronic Disease Prevalence in the U.S. Sociodemographic and Variations by Zip Code Tabulation Area. Preventing Chronic Disease. CDC. 2024, February 29.

18. Southwick, Ron, Physician Shortage Could Reach 86,000 AAMC Projects. Chief HealthCare Executive. 2024, March 22.

19. Top 5 Reasons Why Physicians Are Leaving Their Jobs in 2023; Based on a Survey of 1,639 Doctors. Physician On Fire. 2023, September 19.

20. Kim, Abraham. Four Out Of Five Doctors Are Overworked. Most Are Looking For A Change. 2024, March 25.

21. Physician Workforce: Projections 2021-2036. HRSA Health Workforce. National Center for Health Workforce Analysis. 2023, October.

22. Gao, J, Moran, E., Grimm, R, Toporek, A, Ruser, C. The Effect of Primary Care Visits on Total Patient Care Cost: Evidence From The Veteran's Health Administration, J. Primary Care Community Health. 2022 Dec. 23, 13121501319221141792.

23. Rosenthal, Elisabeth. The Shrinking Number of Primary Care Physicians Is Reaching a Tipping Point. KFF Health News. 2023, September 8.

24. Rae, M, Claxton G, Panchal N, Levitt. Tax Subsidies for Private Health Insurance. KFF. 2014, October 27.

25. Kowalczyk, G, Harden, S. D, Physician Customary Charges and Medicare Payment Experience, Study Findings. Special Report. Health Care Financing Review. Winter 1991, Volume 13, Number 2, p.57-73.

26. Thought Leadership Team. What Are Relative Value Units (RVUs)? AAPC, 2023, December 18.

27. Linzer, M, Bitton, A, Tu, Shin-Ping, Plews-Ogan, M, Schwartz, M.D, The End of the 15-20 Minute Primary Care Visit. J. Gen. Inter. Med. 2015 Apr 22;30(11):1584-1586.

28. The Death of the 15 Minute Visit. Defiant Direct Primary Care.

29. Cubanski, Juliette, Neuman, Tricia. FAQs on Medicare Financing and Trust Fund Solvency. KFF. 2024, May 29.

30. Budget Basics: Medicare. Home. Peter G. Peterson Foundation, 2024, May 20.

31. Sullivan, Kip. Medicare Advantage is a Money Grab by Big Insurers. Minnesota Reformer. 2023, November 3.

32. Berwick, Donald M, MD, MPP, Salve Lucrum: The Existential Threat of Greed in U.S. Health Care," JAMA. 2023: 329(8):629-630.

33. Berg, Sara, MS. What Doctors Wish Patients Knew About Prior Authorization. AMA News Wire. 2023, September 11.

34. How Insurers Deny Legitimate Health Insurance Claims, McKinnon Law Group.

35. Medicare Non-Covered Services, AAFP

36. Sunny Naipaul, Fortune 500 List: The Top 10 Companies Dominating Business, Fortune, 2024, March 8.

37. The Prices That Commercial Health Insurers and Medicare Pay for Hospitals and Physician Services", Congressional Budget Office, 2022, January 20.

38. Lopez, E, Neuman, T, Jacobson, G, Levitt, L, How Much More Than Medicare Do Private Insurers Pay? A Review of the Literature. Medicare. KFF. 2020, April 15.

39. Cubanski, Juliette, Neuman, Tricia. What to Know About Medicare Spending and Financing. Medicare. KFF. 2023, January 19.

40. Kagan, Julia. Unfair Claims Practice: What It Is, How It Works; Examples. Investopedia. 2024, January 23.

41. Greg Daugherty, National Association of Insurance Commissioners (NAIC) Defined. Investopedia. 2022, July 18.

42. Lipschutz, D. Medicare Advantage Plans Under Scrutiny by Department of Justice and Office of Inspector General. Center for Medicare Advisory 2024, February 29.

43. Clemons, Jeffrey PhD., Verger, Stan, PhD., Repeal of the Medicare Sustainable Growth Rate: Direct and Indirect Consequences. Policy Forum. Nov. 2015. AMA Journal of Ethics

44. O'Reilly, Kevin B. Latest Proposed Cut-2.8% -Shows Need for Medicare Pay Reform, AMA News Wire, 2024, July 10.

45. Podkul, Cezary, Representatives Propose Ban on Insurers Charging Doctors a Fee To Be Paid Electronically, Propublica 2023, December 12.

46. 2023 Employer Health Benefits Survey. Health Costs. KFF 2023, October 18.

47. Ortaliza, J, McGough, M, Salaga, M, Amin, Krufika, Cox, Cynthia. How Much and Why 2024 Premiums Are Expected to Grow in Affordable Care Act Market Places. Health Spending. Health System Tracker. Peterson KFF.

48. Nineteen Surgical Organizations Strongly Oppose CMS' Plan to Implement the G2211 Code. Advocacy News. ACS. American College of Surgeons. 2023, July 26.

49. Golinkin, Web. Primary Care: Why It's Important And How to Increase Access To It. Business. Forbes. 2024, February 23.

50. Robertson, Rachel. Is Healthcare Consolidation Fueling the Physician Burnout Crisis? Medphage Today. 2024, September 19.

51. Kane, Carol K. PhD., Policy Research Perspectives. Recent Changes in Physician Practice Arrangements: Shifts Away From Private Practice and Towards Larger Practice Size Continue Through 2022.

52. Smith, Timothy M. 3 Top Reasons Why Doctors Are Selling Their Practices to Hospitals. AMA. Private Practices. 2023, August 29.

53. Bendix, Jeff. The Consequences for Administrative Burdens. Doctors in Private Practice Continues to Dwindle. Medial Economics. 2024, February 1.

54. Grossman, Dan. Large Corporations Buying Up Primary Care Practices at Rapid Pace. Science and Tech. Scripps News. 2023, June 7.

55. Insurer-Owned Clinics Are on the Rise. Applied Health Analytics

56. Corporate Greed in Health Care: A Metastasizing Disease, Community Catalyst. 2024 June 5.

57. Li, Mitchell, Konda, Sailesh, McNamara, Robert. Excessive Corporate Control in Mediciine. Health Justice Monitor. PHNP. 2023 October

58. Landman, MD, Karen. The Profit-Obsessed Monster Destroying American Emergency Rooms, Private Equity Decimated Emergency Care in the United States—Without You Even Noticing It. Vox. 2024, October 3.

59. Fiore, Kristina. Staffing Firm Can't Pay It's Doctors. Special Reports. Medphage Today. 2024, November 1.

60. Schulte, F, Donald, D, Dunkin E, Medicare Advantage Billing Errors Cost Taxpayer Billions. Investigations. NBC News

61. Schulte, Fred. Medicare Advantage's Cost to Taxpayers Has Soared in Recent Years, Research Finds. KFF Health News. Shots. Health News from NPR. 2021, November 1

62. Schulte, Fred. Medicare Advantage Lobbying Steamrolls Congress. Investigating Inequality. The Center for Public Integrity 2014, June 10.

63. The Profitability of Health Insurance Companies. The Council of Economic Advisors. March 2018.

64. Blase, Brian. The ACA Is Making Health Insurers Much Richer. Paragon Health Institute. 2024, March 20.

65. Meller, Abbey, Ahmed, Hauwa. How Big Pharma Reaps Profits While Hurting Everyday Americans. Report. CAP 20. 2019, August 30.

66. Smith, Timothy M. What's The Difference Between Physicians and Nurse Practitioners? Scope of Practice. AMA. 2023, November 22.

67. The Big Question: Will Nurse Practitioners Replace Physicians? NP HUB. 2024, September 7.

68. Bernard, MD, Rebekah. Will Feds Put Final Nail in Coffin of Physician-Led Primary Care? Medical Economics. 2024, February 18.

69. Claxton, G, Rae M. Winger A. Employer-Sponsored Health Insurance 101. KFF. 2024, May 28.

70. Munira Z, Gunja, Evan D, Williams II, R. D. U.S. Health Care From A Global Perspective 2022; Accelerated Spending, Worsening Outcomes, Improving Health Care Quality. The Commonwealth Fund. 2023, January 31.

71. Wager, E, Telesford, I, Rakshit, S, Kuraniand, N, Cox, C. How Does the Quality of the U.S. Health System Compare to Other Countries? Quality of Care. Healthy System Tracker. Peterson KFF. Physicians Advocacy Institute. PAI Avalere Report on Physician Employment

Trends and Acquisition of Medical Practices: 2019-2023 April 2024 (https://www.physiciansadvocacyinstitute.org/PAI Research, PAI-Avalere-Study-on-PhysicianEmployment-Practice-Ownership-Trends-2019-2023)

72. Terry, Ken. Corporate Takeover Has Not Been Good For Healthcare. 4 Sight Health. 2024, August 13.

73. Schulte, Fred. Some Medicare Advantage Plans Overcharged the Government by Billions of Dollars and Got Away With It. Health. The Center for Public Integrity. 2015, December 18.

74. Schulte, Fred. Fraud and Billing Mistakes Cost Medicare-And Tax-payers-Tens of Billions Last Year. Health. The Center for Public Integrity. 2017, July 19.

75. Schulte, Fred. Justice Department Joins Suit Alleging Massive Medicare Fraud by United Health. Health. The Center for Public Integrity. 2017, March 28.

76. Tong, Noah. United Health, CVS and Humana Increasingly Deploy AI and Deny Post-Acute Care Claims, Senate Report Finds. Fierce Healthcare. 2024, October 17.

77. Frieden, Joyce. Stop the Medicare Payment Cut and Pass a Permanent Fix, House Members Urge Leaders. MedPage Today. 2024, October 15.

78. Steinwald, B, Ginsburg, Paul B, Brandt, C, Lee, S, Patel, K. We Need More Primary Care Physicians: Here's Why and How. Commentary. B. 2019, July 8.

79. Reed, Elodie. Randolph Hospital to Hold Forum About It's Future, Cites 'Broken Trust' With Consultant's Report. Vermont Public. 2024, November 7.

80. Oath of Modern Hippocrates. Current Students. Penn State College of Medicine.

81. Primary Care In Crisis: New Scorecard Reveals Sector Struggling to Meet Demand, Return Physicians and Secure Funding. The Physicians Foundation. 2024, February 28.

82. McCauley, L, Robinson, S.K, Meisnere, M, Phillips Jr., R.L, editors. Implementing High Quality Primary Care: Rebuilding the Foundation of HealthCare, National Academies Press (US). 2021, May 4. National Center for Biotechnology Information, National Library of Medicine.

83. Reasons for Private Insurers to Advocate for a Medicaid Expansion. Center on Budget and Policy Priorities.

84. Levitt, MPP, Larry. Increasingly Privatized Public Health Insurance Programs in the U.S. JAMA Health Forum. JAMA Network. 2023, March 30.

85. Ortaliza, J, Biniek, J. F, Hinton, E, Neuman, I, Rudowitz, R, Cox, C. Health Insurer Financial Performance in 2023. Medicare. KFF. 2024, July 2.

86. Geruso, Michael . Layton, Timothy. Upcoding: Evidence From Medicare on Squishy Risk Adjustment. J. Polit. Econ. 2020 Jan 29; (213) 984-1026

87. Glied, Sherry, Chakraborty, Ougni. How the Affordable Care Act Has Affected Health Coverage for Young Men with Higher Incomes. Issue Brief. Commonwealth Fund. April 2018.

88. Lukens, Gidgeon. Health Insurance Costs Will Rise Steeply if Premium Tax Credit Improvements Expire. Health. Center on Budget and Policy Priorities. 2024, June 4.

89. Reno, Jamie. Why You Might See a Nurse Practitioner and Not a Doctor at Your Urgent Care Clinic. Health News. Healthline. 2019, November 4.

90. Benfort, Holly. The Difference Between Direct Primary Care and Concierge Medicine. Health Benefits. People Keep. 2024, November 7.

91. Turner, Terry, Edited by Chowdhury, Lamia, 49+ US Medical Bankruptcy Statistics for 2023, Retire Guide, October 20.2023.

92. Sahni, Nikhil R. M.B.A., M.P.A. I.D., Carrus, Brandon M.Sc. Artificial Intelligence in U.S. Health Care Delivery, N Engl J. Med 2023;389:348-58

93. Zhu, Jan M. M.D., M.P.P., M.S.H.P., Rooke-Ley, Hayden, J.D. and Brown, Erin Fuse, J.D., M.P.H., A Doctrine In Name Only—Strenghthening Prohibitions Against the Corporate Practice of Medicine, N Engl J. Med 2023;389:965-968

94. Blumenthal, D. Gruras, E.D. Shah, A. Gunza, M.Z, Williams II. R.D. Mirror, Mirror 2024: A Portrait of the Failing U.S. Health System, The Commonwealth Fund, September 19,2024

95. The Best Healthcare in the World: Country Rankings. Global Health Insurance, International Citizens Insurance, January 10,2025.

96. Tikkanen, R., Osborn, R. Mossialos, E. Dordjevic, A. Wharton, G. A. Japan International Health Care System Profiles, The Commonwealth Fund, June 5, 2020

THE DECIMATION OF U.S. HEALTHCARE

Book Description

This book describes the evolution of the complex problems facing the U.S. Healthcare System. It elaborates on the greed of third party health insurers, private equity and pharmaceutical giants that have greatly contributed to the decline of U.S. healthcare as well as the complicit nature of lawmakers who have allowed this to happen. The book also describes how the U.S. is accepting a gradual replacement of physicians with non-physician practitioners which significantly lowers the quality of health care rendered. Finally, the book gives solutions to the problem, which calls for monumental change. The results will be better for patients as well as for their caregivers.

www.ingramcontent.com/pod-product-compliance
Lightning Source LLC
Chambersburg PA
CBHW080522030426
42337CB00023B/4600